Plant Based Diet in 30 Minutes

77 Easy Recipes for Busy People

Simple Steps to Create Your Meal Plan

Creative Spun

interim quality. Trademarks that are mentioned are done without written consent and can in no way be considered an endorsement from the trademark holder.

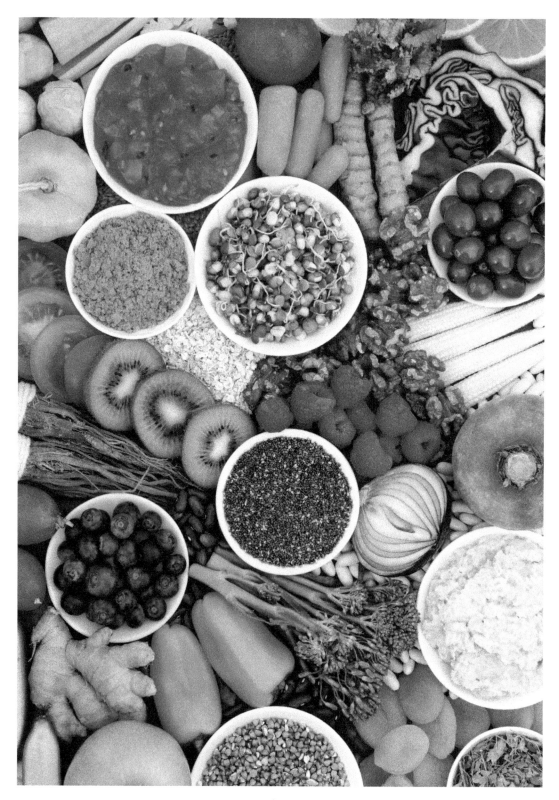

Table of Content

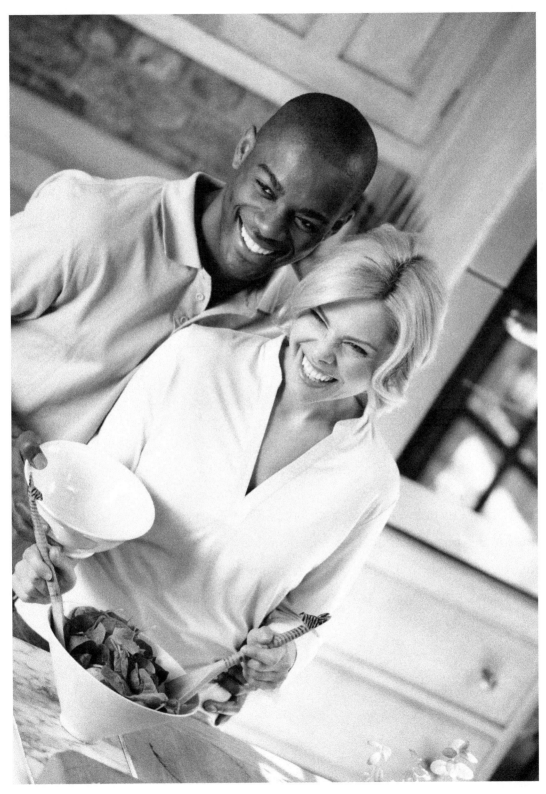

CHAPTER ONE

INTRODUCTION TO PLANT BASED DIET LIFE

Choosing to live a plant-based lifestyle is one of the most important decisions you will ever make. Plant-based diets contain lots of fresh vegetables and fruits, along with nuts, seeds, and whole-grains. There are massive amounts of food just waiting for you to discover them and how delicious they really can be. And you will be leaving behind all of the saturated fats and other toxic substances that are holding back your health now.

It really should not be thought of as a diet plan or a manner of eating because deciding to 'go vegan' will affect all the parts of your life. It will dictate what you buy at the grocery store, where you go to eat out, and may even dictate who you decide to hang out with in your private life.

Research shows that plant-based eating is related to healthy weight management, lower mortality risk, and lower heart disease risk. It is also related to hypertension prevention and treatment, high cholesterol, and lower risk of certain cancers.

Therefore, let us take a journey together as I be your food guide, taking you through some of the basis of the plant-based diets, the health benefits, the nutritional constituents and how it is of great importance to human system, and the incredible plant-based and vegan recipes that you can practice on your own at your convenience.

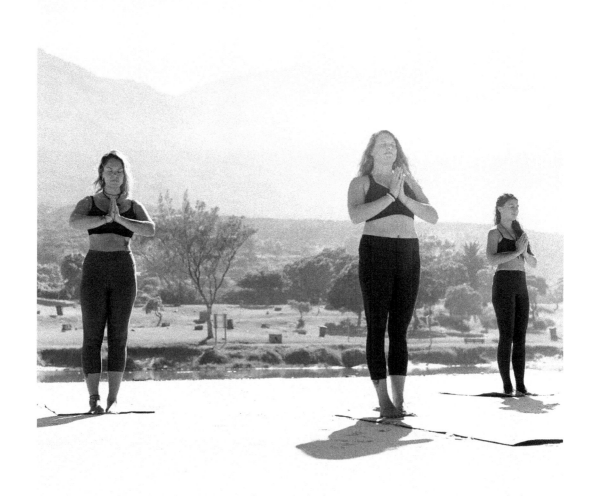

CHAPTER TWO

BASICS ABOUT PLANT BASED DIET AND THE BENEFITS TO YOUR HEALTH

The plant is a good source of closely all the nutrients required by the human body. Plant based diets include fruits, vegetables, nuts, whole grain, and legumes. These are basically plant based foods. With the realization of the various health benefits attributed to plant proteins, people have shifted from consuming animal foods to plant-based foods. Plant based diet includes all unprocessed plant foods. It excludes the consumption of processed foods such as pasta and sugars. It excludes processed fruit juices, milk and milk products, all forms of meat (white and red), and eggs.

FOODS TO AVOID WHEN ON A PLANT BASED DIET

Avoid eating processed foods such as pasta and canned foods. Instead, go for fresh and whole foods. Processed foods are low in their fiber content; they also have other additives such as sugar, salt, preservatives, excess oils, and fats. These foods are linked to the development of chronic illnesses such as cancer, diabetes, hypertension, kidney disease, and heart problems, among others. These foods are also a significant contributor to obesity and weight challenges.

Plant based diet excludes all animal products such as eggs, milk products, poultry, red meat, fish, and any other foods obtained from animals. Animal products are linked to the development of cancers in the human body, especially the heme iron contained in red meat. When animal products are cooked up to certain temperatures, they emit carcinogenic compounds that lead the development of cancer cells. These foods are also a major contributor to weight gain. Research has shown that it is rather a difficulty to watch weight while still on animal products.

Animal related foods are also high in their fat contents and have zero fiber. Consumption of animal products leads to heart problems and hypertension as a result of clogged blood vessels. Their low fiber content makes it a cause of stomach problems such as indigestion and diarrhea.

Avoid the consumption of fast foods such as fries, burgers, cakes, ice cream, and pizza, among others. Fast foods have contents such as processed sugars and high sodium content, high fat content. These foods induce cravings in your body that lead to excessive eating and obesity. The foods are also very unhealthy as they contribute to increased risk of chronic illnesses such as cancer, hypertension, diabetes, heart problems, among others. Fast foods are also low in their nutrient content. Being addictive, when a person forms a habit of consuming fast foods, their bodies go low on some essential nutrients such as vitamins and minerals. They also contain additives that you do not want to put in your bodies due to their toxic nature

FOODS YOU SHOULD BE EATING AS INDIVIDUAL ON A PLANT-BASED DIET

It is of a great essence to state the things you should be eating in a plant-based diet after stating the one you shouldn't eat.

Therefore, here are the things to eat or to look out for to eat when on plant-based diet and they include the following:

- Veggies: spinach, potatoes, kale, squash, cauliflower, and tomatoes
- Legumes: lentils, chickpeas, beans, peas, and peanuts
- Nut butters and nuts
- Whole grains like quinoa, brown rice, barley, and oats

- Tempeh or tofu
- Seeds
- Plant-based oils
- Herbs
- Spices
- Fruits

Any kind of unsweetened beverage like sparkling water, coffee, and tea

HEALTH BENEFITS ASSOCIATED WITH PLANT BASED DIETS

Plant foods offer a wide range of advantages over animal foods. They are scientifically recommended for healthy living as they promote a person's wellbeing. By eating plant-based foods, a person is able to reduce the risk of certain illnesses and avoid problems associated with overweight/obesity.

Plant foods are advantageous in their low fat and calorie load. They are also dense in their protein content. Proteins are excellent in helping a person watch weight as they prevent the gaining of body fat. By consuming plant proteins, a person produces more weight limiting hormones. Proteins also help in weight reduction by reducing the feelings of hunger while at the same time increasing the metabolic rate of the body.

By consuming plant products, a person reduces the risk of being overweight. Plants offer excellent sources of fiber, antioxidants, minerals, and vitamins. Plant foods are mainly high in fiber which is helpful in digestion as it limits the quantity of sugars absorbed in the digestion process. The fiber in plant foods is also helpful in reducing cholesterol by preventing the absorption of fats in the foods we take. Fiber also helps in preventing constipation in enhancing the digestion of foods. It helps in the stimulation of the various digestive organs to produce important digestive juices. Enough intake of dietary fiber prolongs the amount of time food takes to move through the canal, increasing the absorption of minerals and vitamins in the food. It also prevents diarrhea and excessive hardening of stool.

Research has also confirmed that people who take foods high in fiber are at a lower risk of gaining weight. By consuming foods high in fiber, a person reduces the chances of developing type 2 diabetes. The reason behind the fiber preventing the occurrence of type 2 diabetes is the ability of the fiber to reduce the amounts of sugar the body absorbs maintaining a healthy blood sugar level.

It is also attributed to lowered cholesterol and reduced risk of developing heart disease. The fiber in the digestive system also clumps fats reducing the rate at which they are digested and absorbed in the body. Healthy bacteria in the gut thrive on soluble fiber. The bacteria microbiome feeds on the remains of fermented fiber in the digestive system. These bacteria help in the production of short-chain fatty-acids that help in reducing cholesterol in the body. The short chain fatty-acids also promote good health by reducing inflammation in the body. Inflammation is a risky condition linked to the development of serious illnesses such as cancer among others.

Plant foods reduce the risk of cancers, such as colorectal cancer. While animal foods are found to increase the risk of cancer, plants contain phytochemicals and antioxidants that reduce the risk of developing cancer while at the same time fighting the progress of cancer cells. The fiber found in plant foods is also helpful in detoxification of the body. The detoxification process is aided by both soluble and insoluble fiber. The soluble fiber absorbs the excess hormones and toxins within the body, preventing them from being taken up by the cells. Insoluble fiber works by preventing the absorptions of toxins found in the foods we consume from the digestive tract. It also increases the time which food takes to go through the digestive tract. The process is said to reduce the body's demands for more food. The soluble fiber also stimulates the production of certain components that reduce the feelings of hunger which include peptide YY, peptide-1, and cholecystokinin.

When a person is on a plant-based diet, they cut on their consumption of processed foods and refined sugars that are harmful to the body. These sugars promote weight gain by increased food cravings and the production of certain hormones that induce the body to crave for food. These sugars and other additives found in processed food also increase the risk of cancer and among other illnesses.

Plant foods are also rich in certain components that are found to possess anti-oxidation properties while also working in reducing cholesterol levels in the body. These components are polyphenols, such as flavonoids, stilbenoids, and lignans. For instance, green tea, which is most commonly used for its anti-oxidation properties is rich in (epigallocatechin gallate) a flavonoid responsible for the production of the fat burning hormone.

Another beauty of eating plant foods is that you worry less about overeating. The plant foods contain limited calories and negligible levels of harmful fats. According to research, persons who eat plant foods live longer as compared to those that feed on animal foods. Plants foods not only improve the quality of life by protecting a person from illnesses but also lower the risk of early deaths resulting from these illnesses and health conditions.

The benefits of plant-based diet are not limited to the health and fitness only. It is a complete package of ultimate benefits that prolong in society and help each aspect of the society to grow better. Since the diet is all about plants, it means one needs to have fresh vegetables and fruits available in surroundings. Moreover, it enhances the consumption and utilization of all the products and bi-products

Plant based foods are also friendly to the environment. Eating plant foods encourages the planting of more plants to give more foods that protect the ozone layer by absorbing excess harmful carbon dioxide from the atmosphere. Plants based diet discourages the industrial practices associated with processing foods. These practices promote the release of harmful gases into the atmosphere, and the packaging of the foods makes use of materials that are not environmentally friendly.

Plant based diets saves time and money in the sense that Plant-based foods are not as difficult to prepare as meat-based foods. In fact, you will take less time to prepare an organic meal. When you really need, you can easily put together some healthy ingredients and make a quick salad. Furthermore, you spend less money by preparing food using plant-based ingredients. When you source local and organic products, you end up shelling out less cash for the items that you would like to buy.

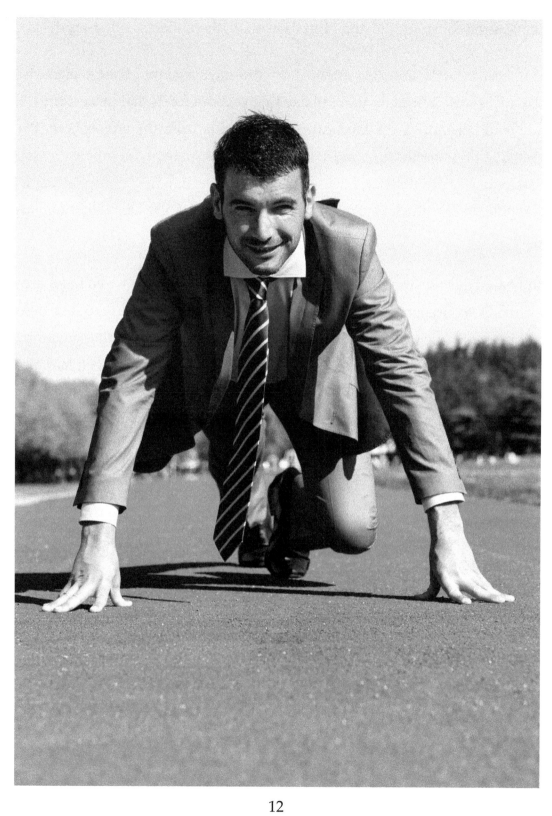

CHAPTER THREE

HOW TO PREPARE FOR YOUR PLANT BASED DIET

Have you ever wondered why you see someone saying they want to take on a new course, new skill, reduce weight, or start a fitness training, or learn how to play golf and you finally see them not achieving this particular goal they set for themselves?

The main reason for failure to achieve this particular goal is found to be as a result of lack of planning. No wonder a saying says that and I quote "when you fail to plan, then obviously you've planned to fail". These words apply to living a plant-based diet life, it is an awesome, beautiful things to say one wants to live a plant-based diet life but once you fail to sit down and strategize about how to go about it, then you will find out later that you aren't achieving this particular goal you set for yourself.

The best way to set yourself up for success for a plant-based diet life is to make a meal plan. When you plan your meals for the week, you will have a good idea of how many meals you need to make and if any events are coming up that you will need to plan for. With a meal plan in hand, you will know exactly what you need to buy for the week and what you are going to eat. With a plan, this leaves very little room for failure. So, how do you make a meal plan? The primary issue with most diets is that they are "cookie-cutter" plans. The truth is, there is no one way to follow a diet. For this reason, learning how to create a meal plan is going to be the best way to stick to your plant-based diet! All you have to do is follow a few simple steps, use some of the delicious recipes provided in this book, and you will be on your merry way of losing, gaining, or even maintaining your weight!

STEPS TO TAKE IN CREATING A MEAL PLAN

- ### *Step One: Nutritional Requirements*

The first step you will need to take when developing a meal plan will be determining how many calories you need. This number will range from person to person as it depends upon your height, weight, sex, age, and activity level. If an individual is on the more active side, they will generally need more calories!

If you want to lose weight on your diet, you will need to cut anywhere from 500-750 calories from your diet. By doing this, you will be able to lose about a pound a week. In general, the average calories per day for an adult can be between 1,600 and 3,200 calories per day. You can find your average and subtract from that number by using an online calculator.

Once you have your calorie recommendation in hand, it is time to find the variety and balance to a proper diet. While following a plant-based diet, this should come relatively easy! Your main focus is going to be on fruits, vegetables, nuts, seeds, and whole-grain foods! Through the proper foods, you will be getting all of your recommended vitamins and minerals.

Knowing your macronutrients is going to be important as you make up your meal plan. As you might already know, there is a common misconception that a plant-based diet means you will lack in protein. We will be going over this a bit later, but all you need to know is that it is not true! While following your new diet, you will still have plenty of protein-rich foods such as beans, legumes, nuts, and soy products. Generally, you will want anywhere from 200-700 of your calories coming from a protein source!

Another critical macronutrient to keep in mind is fat. Unfortunately, fat tends to have a bad representation when it comes to diet. In the market, you will see a ton of products labeled "Non-fat" or "Low-Fat." Spoiler alert: these are just as bad for you! The key here is to realize that there are good fats, and they are necessary for a balanced diet. Generally, you will want to keep your fat intake to 30% or less of your total calories. Good fats can come from sources such as olives, soybeans, and nuts. What it comes down to trans fats and saturated fats; these are the fats that are associated with diabetes and cardiovascular disease.

Just like with fat, carbohydrates are thought of as an "enemy" for individuals who are trying to lose weight. The truth is, carbohydrates play a crucial role in your health! If you want to provide your body with clean energy, it will be important that you choose the right type of carbohydrates. As you create your meal plan, try your best to choose complex carbohydrates. Complex carbohydrates are whole and unprocessed. Some sources of these carbohydrates include legumes, whole-grain bread, vegetables, and some fruits. It is the simple carbohydrates that you will want to avoid! Anything like white bread, white pasta, or white rice has sugars processed and separated from any nutrients.

As you plan out your meals, you will also want to limit your sugar and salt intake. By cutting processed foods, this will happen mostly automatically, but you will still need to be careful of the salt and sugar when you are cooking your own foods. When you have too much sodium in your diet, this leads to fluid retention. Fluid retention is poor because the risk of stroke, heart disease, and high blood pressure can be increased. Generally, you will want to keep sodium to 2,300mg a day or less.

- ***Step Two: Make Your Diet Your Own***

The problem with many diets is that not one size fits all. We all have different goals, different body types, and completely different lifestyles. For this reason, you will need to set your goals and develop a meal plan around that.

First, you will want to decide how much weight you would like to lose or gain, but remember to keep that goal within a reasonable time frame. On average, a person can safely lose about a pound a week. Drastic weight loss is not only unhealthy but also fairly unachievable. Remember to set goals for yourself that are in your reach. By setting attainable goals this can help motivate you to stick to your diet.

Keep in mind that there is no reason you need to change your habits overnight! If you want to lose weight, you will want to make these changes gradually. One of the best ways to do this is by learning how to slow down your meals. Generally, it takes the brain up to twenty minutes to let your body know that you are full. If you consciously eat slower, you will probably feel full quicker!

- ***Step Three: Creating Your Meals***

The final step in creating your own meal plan will be choosing out your meals! If you are just getting started, I highly suggest you try to keep your meal plan as simple as possible. There is absolutely no reason you need to complicate your meals by making separate meals every day of the week!

Instead, consider starting small. If this is your first time, try planning for just breakfast! All you will have to do is take a look at the breakfast recipes provided in this book, choose one or two, and you will be on your way! Once you become more comfortable with the concept of meal planning, you can add more meals to your plan. As you create your meal plans, you will eventually want to include breakfast, lunch, dinner, and some snacks. Luckily, there are many ways to add variety in your meals, so you can really start to get creative!

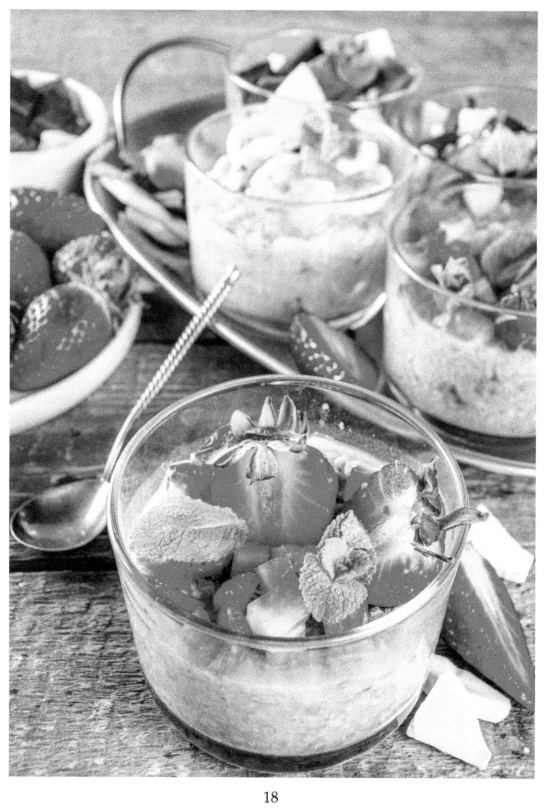

CHAPTER FOUR

PLANT BASED DIET RECIPEE FOR YOUR THREE SQUARED MEALS

BREAKFAST RECIPES

- Fruit and Nut Oatmeal

Preparation Time: 5 minutes

Cooking Time: 10 minutes

Servings: 2

Ingredients:

- ¾ cup rolled oats
- ¼ cup berries, fresh
- ½ ripe banana, sliced
- 2 tablespoons nuts, chopped
- ½ teaspoon cinnamon
- ¼ teaspoon salt
- 2 tablespoons Maple syrup

Directions:

- Put the oats in a small saucepan and add 1½ cups of water. Stir and over high heat, boil. Reduce to low heat and cook for about 5 minutes, or until the water has been absorbed.
- Stir in the cinnamon and add the pinch of salt. Serve in 2 bowls and top each with the chopped fruit and nuts. You can also add a little bit of maple syrup if you want.

Calories 257, Total Fat 6.6g, Saturated Fat 1g, Cholesterol 0mg, Sodium 352mg, Total Carbohydrate 45.7g, Dietary Fiber 5.6g, Total Sugars 17.5g, Protein 6g, Vitamin D 0mcg, Calcium 45mg, Iron 2mg, Potassium 334mg

- Amazing Almond & Banana Granola

Preparation Time: 5 minutes

Cooking Time: 70 minutes

Servings: 8

Ingredients:

- 2 peeled and chopped ripe bananas
- 4 cups of rolled oats
- 1 teaspoon of salt
- 2 cups of freshly chopped and pitted dates
- 1 cup of slivered and toasted almonds
- 1 teaspoon of almond extract

Directions:

- Heat the oven to 275°F.
- With parchment paper, line two 13 x 18-inch baking sheets.
- In an average saucepan, add water, 1 cup and the dates, and boil. On medium heat, cook them for about 10 minutes. The dates will be soft and pulpy. Keep on adding water to the saucepan so that the dates do not stick to the pot.
- After removing the dates from the high temperature, allow them to cool before you blend them with salt, bananas, almond extract.
- You will have a creamy and smooth puree.
- To the oats, add this mixture, and give it a thorough mix.

- Divide the mixture into equal halves and spread over the baking sheets.

- Bake for about 30-40 minutes, and stir every 10 minutes or so.

- You will know that the granola is ready when it becomes crunchy.

- After removing the baking sheets from the cooker, allow them to cool. Then, add the almonds.

- You can store your granola in a container and enjoy it whenever you are hungry.

Nutrition:

Calories 603, Total Fat 14.2g, Saturated Fat 1.5g, Cholesterol 0mg, Sodium 471mg, Total Carbohydrate 112.7g, Dietary Fiber 15.9g, Total Sugars 52.4g, Protein 14.9g, Calcium 116mg, Iron 4mg, Potassium

- Perfect Polenta with a Dose of Cranberries & Pears

Preparation Time: 5 minutes

Cooking Time: 10 minutes

Servings: 4

Ingredients:

- 2 pears freshly cored, peeled, and diced
- 1 cup warm basic polenta
- ¼ cup of brown rice syrup
- 1 teaspoon of ground cinnamon
- 1 cup of dried or fresh cranberries

Directions:

- Warm the polenta in a medium-sized saucepan. Then, add the cranberries, pears, and cinnamon powder.
- Cook everything, stirring occasionally. You will know that the dish is ready when the pears are soft.
- The entire dish will be done within 10 minutes.
- Divide the polenta equally among 4 bowls. Add some pear compote as the last finishing touch.
- Now you can dig into this hassle-free breakfast bowl full of goodness.

Nutrition:

Calories 178, Total Fat 0.3g, Saturated Fat 0g, Cholesterol 0mg, Sodium 17mg, Total Carbohydrate 44.4g, Dietary Fiber 4.9g, Total Sugars 23.8g, Protein 1.9g, Calcium 20mg, Iron 0mg, Potassium 170mg

- Tempeh Bacon Smoked to Perfection

Preparation Time: 5 minutes

Cooking Time: 10 minutes

Servings: 4

Ingredients:

- 3 tablespoons of maple syrup
- 8-ounce package of tempeh
- ¼ cup of soy sauce
- 2 teaspoons of liquid smoke

Directions:

- In a steamer basket, steam the block of tempeh.
- Mix the tamari, maple syrup, and liquid smoke in a medium-sized bowl.
- Once the tempeh cools down, slice into stripes and add to the prepared marinade. Remember: the longer the tempeh marinates, the better the flavor will be. If possible, refrigerate overnight. If not, marinate for at least half an hour.
- In a sauté pan, cook the tempeh on medium-high heat with a bit of the marinade.
- Once the strips get crispy on one side, turn them over so that both sides are evenly cooked.
- You can add some more marinade to cook the tempeh, but they should be properly caramelized. It will take about 5 minutes for each side to cook.

- Enjoy the crispy caramelized tempeh with your favorite dip.

Calories 157, Total Fat 6.2g, Saturated Fat 1.3g, Cholesterol 0mg, Sodium 905mg, Total Carbohydrate 16.6g, Dietary Fiber 0.1g, Total Sugars 9.2g, Protein 11.5g, Calcium 76mg, Iron 2mg, Potassium 299mg

- Quiche with Cauliflower & Chickpea

Preparation Time: 10 minutes

Cooking Time: 30 minutes

Servings: 3

Ingredients:

- ½ teaspoon of salt
- 1 cup of grated cauliflower
- 1 cup of chickpea flour
- ½ teaspoon of baking powder
- ½ zucchini, thinly sliced into half moons
- 1 tablespoon of flax meal
- 1 cup of water
- 4 tbsp fresh rosemary
- ½ teaspoon of Italian seasoning
- ½ freshly sliced red onion

Directions:

- In a bowl, combine all the dry ingredients.
- Chop the onion and zucchini.
- Grate the cauliflower so that it has a rice-like consistency, and add it to the dry ingredients. Now, add the water and mix well.
- Add the zucchini, onion, and rosemary last. You will have a clumpy and thick mixture, but you should be able to spoon it into a tin.

- You can use either a silicone or a metal cake tin with a removable bottom. Now put the mixture in the tin and press it down gently.
- The top should be left messy to resemble a rough texture.
- Bake at 3500 F for about half an hour. You will know your quiche is ready when the top is golden.
- You can serve the quiche warm or cold, as per your preference.

Nutrition:

Calories 280, Total Fat 5.3g, Saturated Fat 0.5g, Cholesterol 1mg, Sodium 422mg, Total Carbohydrate 46.6g, Dietary Fiber 14.2g, Total Sugars 9.4g, Protein 14.7g, Calcium 136mg, Iron 5mg, Potassium 916mg

- Tasty Oatmeal and Carrot Cake

Preparation Time: 5 minutes

Cooking Time: 10 minutes

Servings: 2

Ingredients:

- 1 cup of water
- ½ teaspoon of cinnamon
- 1 cup of rolled oats
- Salt
- ¼ cup of raisins
- ½ cup of shredded carrots
- 1 cup of soy milk
- ¼ teaspoon of allspice
- ½ teaspoon of vanilla extract

Toppings:

- ¼ cup of chopped walnuts
- 2 tablespoons of maple syrup
- 2 tablespoons of shredded coconut

Directions:

- Put a small pot on low heat and bring the non-dairy milk, oats, and water to a simmer.

- Now, add the carrots, vanilla extract, raisins, salt, cinnamon and allspice. You need to simmer all of the ingredients, but do not forget to stir them. You will know that they are ready when the liquid is fully absorbed into all of the ingredients (in about 7-10 minutes).
- Transfer the thickened dish to bowls. You can drizzle some maple syrup on top or top them with coconut or walnuts.
- This nutritious bowl will allow you to kickstart your day.

Nutrition:

Calories 442, Total Fat 15.5g, Saturated Fat 2.7g, Cholesterol 0mg, Sodium 384mg, Total Carbohydrate 66.3g, Dietary Fiber 7.9g, Total Sugars 29g, Protein 13.6g, Vitamin D 1mcg, Calcium 224mg, Iron 5mg, Potassium 520mg

- Almond Butter Banana Overnight Oats

Preparation Time: 5 minutes

Cooking Time: 10 minutes

Servings: 2

Ingredients:

- ½ cup rolled oats
- 1 cup almond milk
- ½ oz chia seeds
- ¼ teaspoon vanilla extract
- ½ teaspoon ground cinnamon
- 1 tablespoon honey
- 1 banana, sliced
- ½ oz almond butter

Instructions:

- Take a large bowl and add the oats, milk, chia seeds, vanilla, cinnamon and honey.
- Stir to combine then divide half of the mixture between two bowls.
- Top with the banana and peanut butter then add the remaining mixture.
- Cover then pop into the fridge overnight.
- Serve and enjoy.

Calories 789, Total Fat 60.1g, Saturated Fat 28.1g, Cholesterol 0mg, Sodium 121mg, Total Carbohydrate 49.4g, Dietary Fiber 14.9g, Total Sugars 22.1g, Protein 20g, Vitamin D 0mcg, Calcium 234mg, Iron 4mg, Potassium 638mg

- Vegan Mango Almond Milkshake

Preparation Time: 4 minutes

Cooking Time: 5 minutes

Servings: 1

Ingredients:

- 1 ripe mango, pulp
- ¾ cup almond milk, unsweetened
- ½ cup Ice

Instructions:

- Grab your blender, add the ingredients and whizz until smooth.
- Serve and enjoy.

Nutrition:

Calories 232, Total Fat 3.9g, Saturated Fat 0.5g, Cholesterol 0mg, Sodium 142mg, Total Carbohydrate 51.8g, Dietary Fiber 6.1g, Total Sugars 45.9g, Protein 3.5g, Vitamin D 1mcg, Calcium 266mg, Iron 1mg, Potassium 708mg

- Peach & Chia Seed Breakfast Parfait

Preparation Time: 5 minutes

Cooking Time: 10 minutes

Servings: 4

Ingredients:

- ½ oz chia seeds
- 1 tablespoon pure maple syrup
- 1 cup coconut milk
- 1 teaspoon ground cinnamon
- 3 medium peaches, diced small
- 2/3 cup granola

Instructions:

- Find a small bowl and add the chia seeds, maple syrup and coconut milk.
- Stir well then cover and pop into the fridge for at least one hour.
- Find another bowl, add the peaches and sprinkle with the cinnamon. Pop to one side.
- When it's time to serve, take two glasses and pour the chia mixture between the two.
- Sprinkle the granola over the top, keeping a tiny amount to one side to use to decorate later.
- Top with the peaches and top with the reserve granola and serve.

Calories 261, Total Fat 25.5g, Saturated Fat 14.5g, Cholesterol 0mg, Sodium 20mg, Total Carbohydrate 40.8g, Dietary Fiber 8.2g, Total Sugars 23.6g, Protein 9.1g, Vitamin D 0mcg, Calcium 73mg, Iron 3mg, Potassium 618mg

- Avocado Toast with White Beans

Preparation Time: 4 minutes

Cooking Time: 6 minutes

Servings: 4

Ingredients:

- ½ cup canned white beans, drained and rinsed
- 2 teaspoons tahini paste
- 2 teaspoons lemon juice
- ½ teaspoon salt
- ½ avocado, peeled and pit removed
- 4 slices whole grain bread, toasted
- ½ cup grape tomatoes, cut in half

Instructions:

- Grab a small bowl and add the beans, tahini, ½ the lemon juice and ½ the salt. Mash with a fork.
- Take another bowl and add the avocado and the remaining lemon juice and salt. Mash together.
- Place your toast onto a flat surface and add the mashed beans, spreading well.
- Top with the avocado and the sliced tomatoes then serve and enjoy.

Calories 245, Total Fat 8g, Saturated Fat 1.3g, Cholesterol 0mg, Sodium 431mg, Total Carbohydrate 33.8g, Dietary Fiber 10g, Total Sugars 3.3g, Protein 11g, Vitamin D 0mcg, Calcium 77mg, Iron 4mg, Potassium 642mg

- Homemade Granola

Preparation Time: 5 minutes

Cooking Time: 1 hour 15 minutes

Servings: 7

Ingredients:

- 5 cups rolled oats
- 1 cup almonds, slivered
- ¾ cup coconut, shredded
- ¾ tsp salt
- ¼ cup coconut oil
- ½ cup maple syrup

Directions:

- Preheat oven to 250°F.
- Mix all ingredients in a large bowl.
- Spread granola evenly on two rimmed sheet pans.
- Bake at 250°F for 1 hour 15 minutes, stirring every 20-25 min.
- Let cool in pans, and serve.

Nutrition Facts Per Serving:

Calories 456, Total Fat 21.3g, Saturated Fat 10.5g, Cholesterol 0mg, Sodium 255mg, Total Carbohydrate 58.9g, Dietary Fiber 8.4g, Total Sugars 15.1g, Protein 10.8g, Vitamin D 0mcg, Calcium 82mg, Iron 4mg, Potassium 387mg

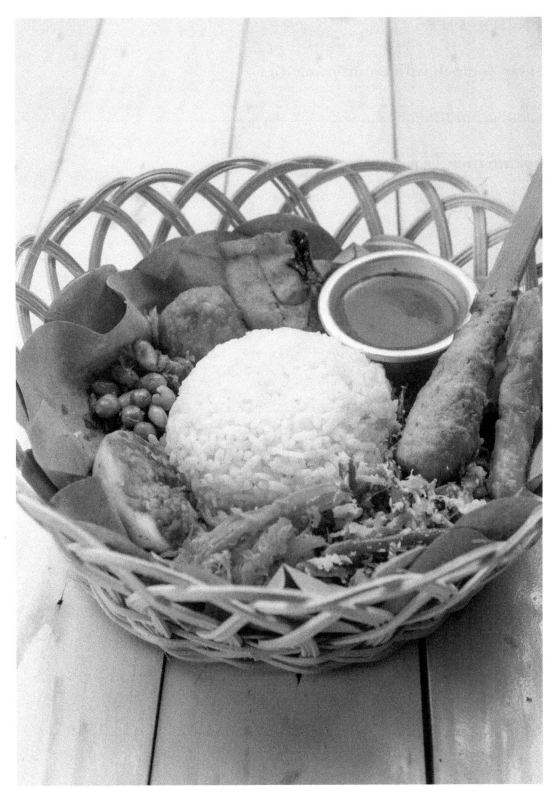

LUNCH RECIPES

- Satay Tempeh with Cauliflower Rice

Preparation time: 60 minutes

Cooking time: 15 minutes

Servings: 4

Ingredients:

- ¼ cup water
- 4 tbsp. peanut butter
- 3 tbsp. low sodium soy sauce
- 2 tbsp. coconut sugar
- 1 garlic clove, minced
- 1 tbsp ginger, minced
- 2 tsp. rice vinegar
- 1 tsp. red pepper flakes
- 4 tbsp. olive oil
- 2 8-oz. packages tempeh, drained
- 2 cups cauliflower rice
- 1 cup purple cabbage, diced
- 1 tbsp. sesame oil
- 1 tsp. agave nectar

Directions:

- Take a large bowl, combine all the ingredients for the sauce, and then whisk until the mixture is smooth and any lumps have dissolved.
- Cut the tempeh into ½-inch cubes and put them into the sauce, stirring to make sure the cubes get coated thoroughly.
- Place the bowl in the refrigerator to marinate the tempeh for up to 3 hours.
- Before the tempeh is done marinating, preheat the oven to 400°F.
- Spread the tempeh out in a single layer on a baking sheet lined with parchment paper or lightly greased with olive oil.
- Bake the marinated cubes until browned and crisp—about 15 minutes.
- Heat the cauliflower rice in a saucepan with 2 tablespoons of olive oil over medium heat until it is warm.
- Rinse the large bowl with water, and then mix the cabbage, sesame oil, and agave together.
- Serve a scoop of the cauliflower rice topped with the marinated cabbage and cooked tempeh on a plate or in a bowl and enjoy. Or, store for later.

Nutrition:

Calories 554, Total Fat 38.8g, Saturated Fat 7.1g, Cholesterol 0mg, Sodium 614mg, Total Carbohydrate 32.3g, Dietary Fiber 2.1g, Total Sugars 13.9g, Protein 28.1g, Vitamin D 0mcg, Calcium 140mg, Iron 5mg, Potassium 655mg

- Teriyaki Tofu Wraps

Preparation time: 30 minutes

Cooking time: 15 minutes

Servings: 3

Ingredients:

- 14-oz. drained, package extra firm tofu
- 1 small white onion, diced
- 1 cup chopped pineapple
- ¼ cup soy sauce
- 2 tbsp. sesame oil
- 1 garlic clove, minced
- 1 tsp. coconut sugar
- 4 large lettuce leaves
- 1 tbsp. roasted sesame seeds
- ¼ tsp Salt
- ¼ tsp pepper

Directions:

- Take a medium-sized bowl and mix the soy sauce, sesame oil, coconut sugar, and garlic.
- Cut the tofu into ½-inch cubes, place them in the bowl, and transfer the bowl to the refrigerator to marinate, up to 3 hours.
- Meanwhile, cut the pineapple into rings or cubes.

- After the tofu is adequately marinated, place a large skillet over medium heat, and pour in the tofu with the remaining marinade, pineapple cubes, and diced onions; stir.
- Add salt and pepper to taste, making sure to stir the ingredients frequently, and cook until the onions are soft and translucent—about 15 minutes.
- Divide the mixture between the lettuce leaves and top with a sprinkle of roasted sesame seeds.
- Serve right away, or, store the mixture and lettuce leaves separately.

Nutrition:

Calories 247, Total Fat 16.2g, Saturated Fat 2.6g, Cholesterol 0mg, Sodium 1410mg, Total Carbohydrate 16.1g, Dietary Fiber 3.1g, Total Sugars 9g, Protein 13.4g, Vitamin D 0mcg, Calcium 315mg, Iron 4mg, Potassium 371mg

- Tex-Mex Tofu & Beans

Preparation time: 25 minutes

Cooking time: 12 minutes

Servings: 2

Ingredients:

- 1 cup dry black beans
- 1 cup dry brown rice
- 1 14-oz. package firm tofu, drained
- 2 tbsp. olive oil
- 1 small purple onion, diced
- 1 medium avocado, pitted, peeled
- 1 garlic clove, minced
- 1 tbsp. lime juice
- 2 tsp. cumin
- 2 tsp. paprika
- 1 tsp. chili powder
- ¼ tsp Salt
- ¼ tsp pepper

Directions:

- Cut the tofu into ½-inch cubes.
- Heat the olive oil in a large skillet over high heat. Add the diced onions and cook until soft, for about 5 minutes.

- Add the tofu and cook an additional 2 minutes, flipping the cubes frequently.
- Meanwhile, cut the avocado into thin slices and set aside.
- Lower the heat to medium and mix in the garlic, cumin, and cooked black beans.
- Stir until everything is incorporated thoroughly, and then cook for an additional 5 minutes.
- Add the remaining spices and lime juice to the mixture in the skillet. Mix thoroughly and remove the skillet from the heat.
- Serve the Tex-Mex tofu and beans with a scoop of rice and garnish with the fresh avocado.
- Enjoy immediately, or, store the rice, avocado, and tofu mixture separately.

Nutrition:

Calories 1175, Total Fat 46.8g, Saturated Fat 8.8g, Cholesterol 0mg, Sodium 348mg, Total Carbohydrate 152.1g, Dietary Fiber 28.8g, Total Sugars 5.7g, Protein 47.6g, Vitamin D 0mcg, Calcium 601mg, Iron 13mg, Potassium 2653mg

- Vegan Friendly Fajitas

Preparation time: 30 minutes

Cooking time: 19 minutes

Servings: 6

Ingredients:

- 1 cup dry black beans
- 1 large green bell pepper, seeded, diced
- 1 poblano pepper, seeded, thinly sliced
- 1 large avocado, peeled, pitted, mashed
- 1 medium sweet onion, chopped
- 3 large portobello mushrooms
- 2 tbsp. olive oil
- 6 tortilla wraps
- 1 tsp. lime juice
- 1 tsp. chili powder
- 1 tsp. garlic powder
- ¼ tsp. cayenne pepper
- ¼ tsp Salt

Directions:

- Prepare the black beans according to the method.
- Heat 1 tablespoon of olive oil in a large frying pan over high heat.
- Add the bell peppers, poblano peppers, and half of the onions.

- Mix in the chili powder, garlic powder, and cayenne pepper; add salt to taste.
- Cook the vegetables until tender and browned, around 10 minutes.
- Add the black beans and continue cooking for an additional 2 minutes; then remove the frying pan from the stove.
- Add the portobello mushrooms to the skillet and turn heat down to low. Sprinkle the mushrooms with salt.
- Stir/flip the ingredients often, and cook until the mushrooms have shrunk down to half their size, around 7 minutes. Remove the frying pan from the heat.
- Mix the avocado, remaining 1 tablespoon of olive oil, and the remaining onions together in a small bowl to make a simple guacamole. Mix in the lime juice and add salt and pepper to taste.
- Spread the guacamole on a tortilla with a spoon and then top with a generous scoop of the mushroom mixture.
- Serve and enjoy right away, or, allow the prepared tortillas to cool down and wrap them in paper towels to store!

Nutrition:

Calories 429, Total Fat 16.8g, Saturated Fat 3.2g, Cholesterol 0mg, Sodium 627mg, Total Carbohydrate 59.2g, Dietary Fiber 12.7g, Total Sugars 4.2g, Protein 14.8g, Vitamin D 0mcg, Calcium 113mg, Iron 4mg, Potassium 899mg

- Tofu Cacciatore

Preparation time: 45 minutes

Cooking time: 35 minutes

Servings: 3

Ingredients:

- 1 14-oz. package extra firm tofu, drained
- 1 tbsp. olive oil
- 1 cup matchstick carrots
- 1 medium sweet onion, diced
- 1 medium green bell pepper, seeded, diced
- 1 28-oz. can dice tomatoes
- 1 4-oz. can tomato paste
- ½ tbsp. balsamic vinegar
- 1 tbsp. soy sauce
- 1 tbsp. maple syrup
- 1 tbsp. garlic powder
- 1 tbsp. Italian seasoning
- ¼ tsp Salt
- ¼ tsp pepper

Directions:

- Chop the tofu into ¼- to ½-inch cubes.
- Heat the olive oil in a large skillet over medium-high heat.

- Add the onions, garlic, bell peppers, and carrots; sauté until the onions turn translucent, around 10 minutes. Make sure to stir frequently to prevent burning.
- Now add the balsamic vinegar, soy sauce, maple syrup, garlic powder and Italian seasoning.
- Stir well while pouring in the diced tomatoes and tomato paste; mix until all ingredients are thoroughly combined.
- Add the cubed tofu and stir one more time.
- Cover the pot, turn the heat to medium-low, and allow the mixture to simmer until the sauce has thickened, for around 20-25 minutes.
- Serve the tofu cacciatore in bowls and top with salt and pepper to taste, or, store for another meal!

Nutrition:

Calories 319, Total Fat 12g, Saturated Fat 2.1g, Cholesterol 3mg, Sodium 1156mg, Total Carbohydrate 43.1g, Dietary Fiber 10.4g, Total Sugars 27.1g, Protein 17.6g, Vitamin D 0mcg, Calcium 359mg, Iron 5mg, Potassium 961mg

- Portobello Burritos

Preparation time: 50 minutes

Cooking time: 40 minutes

Servings: 4

Ingredients:

- 3 large portobello mushrooms
- 2 medium potatoes
- 4 tortilla wraps
- 1 medium avocado, pitted, peeled, diced
- ¾ cup salsa
- 1 tbsp. cilantro
- ½ tsp salt
- 1/3 cup water
- 1 tbsp. lime juice
- 1 tbsp. minced garlic
- ¼ cup teriyaki sauce

Directions:

- Preheat the oven to 400°F.
- Lightly grease a sheet pan with olive oil (or alternatively, line with parchment paper) and set it aside.
- Combine the water, lime juice, teriyaki, and garlic in a small bowl.
- Slice the portobello mushrooms into thin slices and add these to the bowl.

Allow the mushrooms to marinate thoroughly, for up to three hours.

- Cut the potatoes into large matchsticks, like French fries. Sprinkle the fries with salt and then transfer them to the sheet pan. Place the fries in the oven and bake them until crisped and golden, around 30 minutes. Flip once halfway through for even cooking.

- Heat a large frying pan over medium heat. Add the marinated mushroom slices with the remaining marinade to the pan. Cook until the liquid has absorbed, around 10 minutes. Remove from heat.

- Fill the tortillas with a heaping scoop of the mushrooms and a handful of the potato sticks. Top with salsa, sliced avocados, and cilantro before serving.

- Serve right away and enjoy, or, store the tortillas, avocado, and mushrooms separately for later!

Nutrition:

Calories 391, Total Fat 14.9g, Saturated Fat 3.1g, Cholesterol 0mg, Sodium 1511mg, Total Carbohydrate 57g, Dietary Fiber 10.8g, Total Sugars 5.1g, Protein 11.2g, Vitamin D 0mcg, Calcium 85mg, Iron 3mg, Potassium 956mg

- Mushroom Madness Stroganoff

Preparation time: 30 minutes

Cooking time: 25 minutes

Servings: 4

Ingredients:

- 2 cups gluten-free noodles
- 1 small onion, chopped
- 2 cups vegetable broth
- 2 tbsp. almond flour
- 1 tbsp. tamari
- 1 tsp. tomato paste
- 1 tsp. lemon juice
- 3 cups mushrooms, chopped
- 1 tsp. thyme
- 3 cups raw spinach
- 1 tbsp. apple cider vinegar
- 1 tbsp. olive oil
- ¼ tsp Salt
- ¼ tsp pepper
- 2 tbsp. fresh parsley

Directions:

- Prepare the noodles according to the package instructions.
- Heat the olive oil in a large skillet over medium heat.
- Add the chopped onion and sauté until soft—for about 5 minutes.
- Stir in the flour, vegetable broth, tamari, tomato paste, and lemon juice; cook for an additional 3 minutes.
- Blend in the mushrooms, thyme, and salt to taste, then cover the skillet.
- Cook until the mushrooms are tender, for about 7 minutes, and turn the heat down to low.
- Add the cooked noodles, spinach, and vinegar to the pan and top the ingredients with salt and pepper to taste.
- Cover the skillet again and let the flavors combine for another 8-10 minutes.
- Serve immediately, topped with the optional parsley if desired, or, store and enjoy the stroganoff another day of the week!

Nutrition:

Calories 240, Total Fat 11.9g, Saturated Fat 1.3g, Cholesterol 0mg, Sodium 935mg, Total Carbohydrate 26.1g, Dietary Fiber 4.3g, Total Sugars 4.9g, Protein 9.9g, Vitamin D 189mcg, Calcium 71mg, Iron 4mg, Potassium 463mg

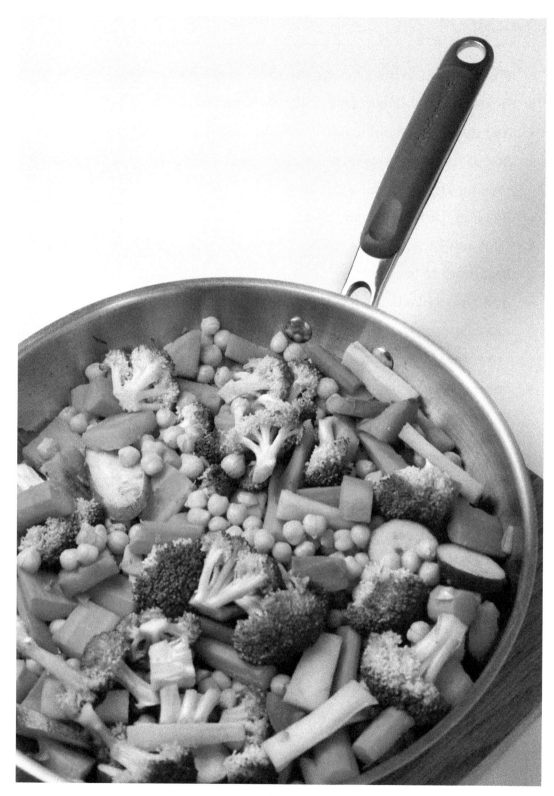

54

DINNER RECIPEE

- Mean bean minestrone

Preparation time: 45 minutes

Servings: 6

Protein content per serving: 9g

Ingredients:

- 1 tablespoon (15 ml) olive oil
- 1/3 cup (80 g) chopped red onion
- 4 cloves garlic, grated or pressed
- 1 leek, white and light green parts, trimmed and chopped (about 4 ounces, or 113 g)
- 2 carrots, peeled and minced (about 4 ounces, or 113 g)
- 2 ribs of celery, minced (about 2 ounces, or 57 g)
- 2 yellow squashes, trimmed and chopped (about 8 ounces, or 227 g)
- 1 green bell pepper, trimmed and chopped (about 8 ounces, or 227 g)
- 1 tablespoon (16 g) tomato paste
- 1 teaspoon dried oregano
- 1 teaspoon dried basil
- ⅓ teaspoon smoked paprika
- '¼ to ¼ teaspoon cayenne pepper, or to taste
- 2 cans (each 15 ounces, or 425 g) diced fire-roasted tomatoes
- 4 cups (940 ml) vegetable broth, more if needed
- 3 cups (532 g) cannellini beans, or other white beans

- 2 cups (330 g) cooked farro, or other whole grain or pasta
- Salt, to taste
- Nut and seed sprinkles, for garnish, optional and to taste

Directions:

- In a large pot, add the oil, onion, garlic, leek, carrots, celery, yellow squash, bell pepper, tomato paste, oregano, basil, paprika, and cayenne pepper. Cook on medium-high heat, stirring often until the vegetables start to get tender, about 6 minutes.
- Add the tomatoes and broth. Bring to a boil, lower the heat, cover with a lid, and simmer 15 minutes.
- Add the beans and simmer another 10 minutes. Add the farro and simmer 5 more minutes to heat the farro.
- Note that this is a thick minestrone. If there are leftovers (which taste even better, by the way), the soup will thicken more once chilled.
- Add extra broth if you prefer a thinner soup and adjust seasoning if needed. Add nut and seed sprinkles on each portion upon serving, if desired.
- Store leftovers in an airtight container in the refrigerator for up to 5 days. The minestrone can also be frozen for up to 3 months.

- Sushi rice and bean stew

Preparation time: 45 minutes

Servings: 6

Ingredients:

For the sushi rice:

- 1 cup (208 g) dry sushi rice, thoroughly rinsed until water runs clear and drained
- 1¾ cups (295 ml) water
- 1 tablespoon (15 ml) fresh lemon juice
- 1 teaspoon toasted sesame oil
- 1 teaspoon sriracha
- 1 teaspoon tamari
- 1 teaspoon agave nectar or brown rice syrup

For the stew:

- 1 tablespoon (15 ml) toasted sesame oil
- 9 ounces (255 g) minced carrot (about 4 medium carrots)
- 1/3 cup (80 g) chopped red onion or ¼ cup (40 g) minced shallot
- 2 teaspoons grated fresh ginger or ⅓ teaspoon ginger powder 4 cloves garlic, grated or pressed
- I½ cups (246 g) cooked chickpeas
- 1 cup (155 g) frozen, shelled edamame
- 3 tablespoons (45 ml) seasoned rice vinegar

- 2 tablespoons (30 ml) tamari
- 2 teaspoons sriracha, or to taste
- 1 cup (235 ml) mushroom-soaking broth
- 2 cups (470 ml) vegetable broth
- 2 tablespoons (36 g) white miso
- 2 tablespoons (16 g) toasted white sesame seeds

Directions:

- To make the sushi rice: combine the rice and water in a rice cooker, cover with the lid, and cook until the water is absorbed without lifting the lid. (alternatively, cook the rice on the stove top, following the directions on the package.) While the rice is cooking, combine the remaining sushi rice ingredients in a large bowl.
- Let the rice steam for 10 minutes in the rice cooker with the lid still on. Gently fold the cooked rice into the dressing. Set aside.
- To make the stew: heat the oil in a large pot on medium-high heat. Add the carrots, onion, ginger, and garlic. Lower the temperature to medium and cook until the vegetables start to get tender, stirring often about 4 minutes.
- Add the chickpeas, edamame, vinegar, tamari, and sriracha. Stir and cook for another 4 minutes. Add the broths, and bring back to a slow boil. Cover with a lid, lower the heat, and simmer for 10 minutes.
- Place the miso in a small bowl and remove 3 tablespoons (45 ml) of the broth from the pot. Stir into the miso to thoroughly combine. Stir the miso mixture back into the pan, and remove from the heat.
- Divide the rice among 4 to 6 bowls, depending on your appetite. Add approximately 1 cup (235 ml) of the stew on top of each portion of rice. Add 1 teaspoon of sesame seeds on top of each serving, and serve immediately.

- If you do not plan on eating this dish in one shot, keep the rice and stew separated and store in the refrigerator for up to 4 days.
- When reheating the stew, do not bring to a boil. Slowly warm the rice with the stew on medium heat in a small saucepan until heated through.

- Giardiniera chili

Preparation time: 35 minutes

Servings: 6

Protein content per serving: 28 g

Ingredients:

- 1 tablespoon (15 ml) neutral-flavored oil
- 1 medium red onion, chopped
- 4 carrots, peeled and minced (9 ounces, or 250 g)
- 2 zucchini, trimmed and minced (11 ounces, or 320 g)
- 4 roma tomatoes, diced (14 ounces, or 400 g)
- 4 cloves garlic, grated or pressed
- 1 tablespoon (8 g) mild to medium chili powder
- 1 teaspoon ground cumin
- ½ teaspoon smoked paprika
- ½ teaspoon liquid smoke
- ¼ teaspoon fine sea salt, or to taste
- ¼ teaspoon cayenne pepper, or to taste
- 2 tablespoons (32 g) tomato paste
- 1 can (15 ounces, or 425 g) diced fire-roasted tomatoes
- ½ cup (120 ml) vegetable broth
- ½ cup (120 ml) mushroom-soaking broth or extra vegetable broth
- 1 can (15 ounces, or 425 g) pinto beans, drained and rinsed
- 1 can (15 ounces, or 425 g) black beans, drained and rinsed
- ½ cup (60 g) nutritional yeast

Directions:

- Heat the oil on medium-high in a large pot and add the onion, carrots, zucchini, tomatoes, and garlic. Cook for 6 minutes, stirring occasionally until the carrots start to get tender. Add the chili powder, cumin, paprika, liquid smoke, salt, cayenne pepper, and tomato paste, stirring to combine. Cook another 2 minutes. Add the diced tomatoes, broths, beans, and nutritional yeast. Bring to a low boil. Lower the heat, cover with a lid, and simmer 15 minutes, stirring occasionally. Remove the lid and simmer for another 5 minutes.
- Serve on top of a cooked whole grain of choice or with your favorite chili accompaniments.
- Leftovers can be stored in an airtight container in the refrigerator for up to 4 days or frozen for up to 3 months.

- Shorba (lentil soup)

Preparation time: 30 minutes

Servings: 6

Protein content per serving: 10 g

Ingredients:

- 1 tablespoon (15 ml) olive oil
- 1 medium onion, minced
- 1 large carrot, peeled and chopped
- 1 fist-size russet potato, cut into small cubes (about 7 ounces, or 198 g)
- 4 large cloves garlic, minced
- 2 teaspoons grated fresh ginger root
- 1 to 2 teaspoons berbere, to taste
- 1/3 teaspoon turmeric
- 1 cup (192 g) brown lentils, picked over and rinsed
- 6 cups (1.4 l) water, more if desired
- 1 tablespoon (16 g) tomato paste
- 1 tablespoon (18 g) vegetable bouillon paste, or 2 bouillon cubes
- Salt and pepper

Directions:

- Heat the oil in a large soup pot over medium heat. Add the onion, carrot, and potato. Cook for 5 to 7 minutes, stirring occasionally until the onions are translucent. Stir in the garlic, ginger, berbere, turmeric, and lentils and cook and stir for 1 minute until fragrant. Add the water, tomato paste, and bouillon. Bring to a boil, and then reduce the heat to a simmer. Cook for 30 minutes, stirring occasionally until the lentils are tender. Taste and adjust the seasonings.

- The whole enchilada

Preparation time: 20 minutes

Servings: 6

Protein content per enchilada: 6 g

For the sauce:

- 2 tablespoons (30 ml) olive oil 1/3 cup (80 g) chopped red onion 4 ounces (113 g) tomato paste
- 1 tablespoon (15 ml) adobo sauce
- 1 tablespoon (8 g) mild to medium chili powder
- 1 teaspoon ground cumin
- 3 cloves garlic, grated or pressed
- ⅓ teaspoon fine sea salt, or to taste
- 2 tablespoons (15 g) whole wheat pastry flour or (16 g) all-purpose flour
- 2 cups (470 ml) water

For the filling:

- 1 protein content per serving teaspoons olive oil
- ⅓ cup (53 g) chopped red onion
- 1 sweet potato, trimmed and peeled, chopped (about 8.8 ounces, or 250 g)
- 1 yellow squash, trimmed and chopped (about 5.3 ounces, or 150 g)
- 2 cloves garlic, grated or pressed
- 1 tablespoon (8 g) nutritional yeast

64

- 1 smoked paprika
- ¼ teaspoon liquid smoke
- Pinch of fine sea salt, or to taste
- 1 (258 g) cooked black beans
- 3 tablespoons (45 ml) enchilada sauce
- 12 to 14 corn tortillas
- 1 recipe creamy cashew sauce
- Chopped fresh cilantro, to taste hot sauce, to taste

Directions:

- To make the sauce: heat the oil on medium heat in a large skillet. Add the onion and cook until fragrant while occasionally stirring, about 2 minutes. Add the tomato paste, adobo sauce, chili powder, cumin, garlic, and salt. Saute for 2 minutes, stirring frequently. Sprinkle the flour on top and cook 2 minutes, stirring frequently. Slowly whisk in the water and cook until slightly thickened, about 6 minutes, frequently whisking to prevent clumps. Remove from the heat and set aside.

To make the filling: heat the oil in a large skillet on medium heat. Add the onion and sweet potato and cook 6 minutes or until the potato starts to get tender, stirring occasionally. Add the squash and garlic and cook for 4 minutes, stirring occasionally. Add the nutritional yeast, paprika, liquid smoke, and salt, stir to combine, and cook for another minute. Add the beans and enchilada sauce and stir to combine. Cover the pan and simmer until the vegetables are completely tender about 4 minutes. Add a little water if the plants stick to the skillet. Adjust the seasonings if needed.

Preheat the oven to 350°f (180°c, or gas mark 4).

Place the sauce in a large shallow bowl. If you aren't using pre-shaped, uncooked tortillas, follow the direction in the recipe notes to soften the tortillas so that they are easier to work with. Ladle about 1/3 cup (80 ml) of enchilada sauce on the bottom of a 9 x 13-inch (23 x 33 cm) baking dish. Dip each tortilla in the sauce to coat only lightly. Don't be too generous and gently scrape off the excess sauce with a spatula; otherwise, you will run out of sauce. Add a scant ¼ cup (about 45 g) of the filling in each tortilla. Fold the tortilla over the filling, rolling like a cigar. Place the enchiladas in the pan, seam side down. Make sure to squeeze them in tight so that there's room in the dish for all of them. Top evenly with the remaining enchilada sauce. Add the creamy cashew sauce consistently on top.

Bake for 20 to 25 minutes or until the top is set, and the enchiladas are heated through. Garnish with cilantro and serve with hot sauce.

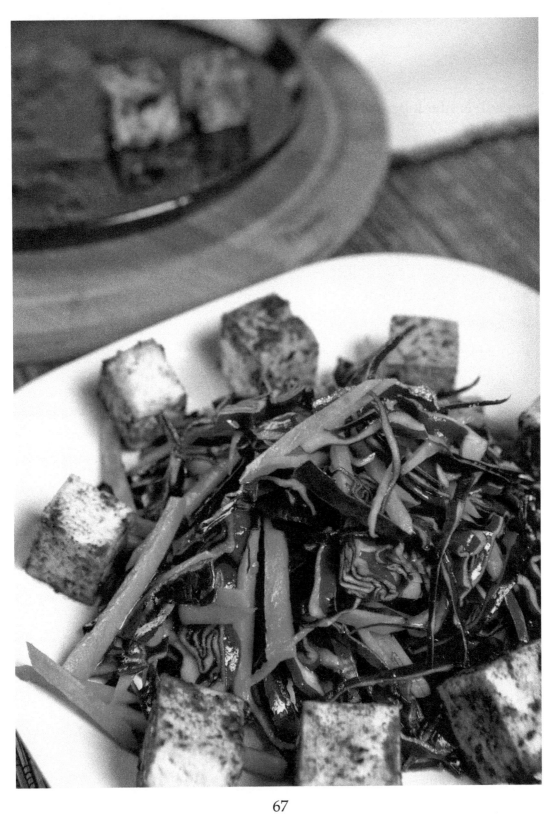

CHAPTER FIVE

MAIN COURSE RECIPES

- Broccoli & black beans stir fry

Preparation time: 60 minutes

Servings: 6

Ingredients:

- 4 cups broccoli florets
- 2 cups cooked black beans
- 1 tablespoon sesame oil
- 4 teaspoons sesame seeds
- 2 cloves garlic, finely minced
- 2 teaspoons ginger, finely chopped
- A large pinch red chili flake
- A pinch turmeric powders
- Salt to taste
- Lime juice to taste (optional)

Direction:

- Steam broccoli for 6 minutes. Drain and set aside.
- Warm the sesame oil in a large frying pan over medium heat. Add sesame seeds, chili flakes, ginger, garlic, turmeric powder, and salt. Sauté for a couple of minutes.
- Add broccoli and black beans and sauté until thoroughly heated.
- Sprinkle lime juice and serve hot.

- Sweet 'n spicy tofu

Preparation time: 45 minutes

Servings: 8

Ingredients:

- 14 ounces extra firm tofu; press the excess liquid and chop into cubes.
- 3 tablespoons olive oil
- 2 2-3 cloves garlic, minced
- 4 tablespoons sriracha sauce or any other hot sauce
- 2 tablespoons soy sauce
- 1/4 cup sweet chili sauce
- 5-6 cups mixed vegetables of your choice (like carrots, cauliflower, broccoli, potato, etc.)
- Salt to taste (optional)

Directions:

- Place a nonstick pan over medium-high heat. Add 1 tablespoon oil. When oil is hot, add garlic and mixed vegetables and stir-fry until crisp and tender. Remove and keep aside.
- Place the pan back on heat. Add 2 tablespoons oil. When oil is hot, add tofu and sauté until golden brown. Add the sautéed vegetables. Mix well and remove from heat.
- Make a mixture of sauces by mixing together all the sauces in a small bowl.
- Serve the stir-fried vegetables and tofu with sauce.

- Eggplant & Mushrooms in Peanut Sauce

Preparation time: 32 minutes

Servings: 6

Ingredients:

- 4 Japanese eggplants cut into 1-inch-thick round slices
- 3/4 pounds of shiitake mu shrooms, stems discarded, halved
- 3 tablespoons smooth peanut butter
- 2 1/2 tablespoons rice vinegar
- 1 1/2 tablespoons soy sauce
- 1 1/2 tablespoons, peeled, fresh ginger, finely grated
- 1 1/2 tablespoons light brown sugar
- Coarse salt to taste
- 3 scallions, cut into 2-inch lengths, thinly sliced lengthwise

Direction:

- Place the eggplants and mushroom in a steamer. Steam the eggplant and mushrooms until tender. Transfer to a bowl.
- To a small bowl, add peanut butter and vinegar and whisk.
- Add rest of the ingredients and whisk well. Add this to the bowl of eggplant slices. Add scallions and mix well and serve hot.

- Green beans stir fry

Preparation time: 30 minutes

Servings: 6-8

Ingredients:

- 1 1/2 pounds of green beans, stringed, chopped into 1 ½-inch pieces
- 1 large onion, thinly sliced
- 4-star anise (optional)
- 3 tablespoons avocado oil
- 1 1/2 tablespoons tamari sauce or soy sauce
- Salt to taste
- 3/4 cup water

Direction:

1. Place a wok over medium heat. Add oil. When oil is heated, add onions and sauté until onions are translucent.
2. Add beans, water, tamari sauce, and star anise and stir. Cover and cook until the beans are tender.
3. Uncover, add salt and raise the heat to high. Cook until the water dries up in the wok. Stir a couple of times while cooking.

- Collard greens 'n tofu

Preparation time: 15 minutes

Servings: 4

Ingredients:

- 2 pounds of collard greens, rinsed, chopped
- 1 cup water
- 1/2 pound of tofu, chopped
- Salt to taste
- Pepper powder to taste
- Crushed red chili to taste

Direction:

- Place a large skillet over medium-high heat. Add oil. When the oil is heated, add tofu and cook until brown.
- Add rest of the ingredients and mix well.
- cook until greens wilts and almost dry.

- Double-garlic bean and vegetable soup

Preparation time: 25 minutes

Servings: 4

Protein content per serving: 21 g

Ingredients:

- 1 tablespoon (15 ml) olive oil
- 1 teaspoon fine sea salt
- 1 (240 g) minced onion 5 cloves garlic, minced
- 2 cups (220 g) chopped red potatoes
- ⅔ cup (96 g) sliced carrots
- Protein content per serving cup (60 g) chopped celery
- 1 teaspoon Italian seasoning blend
- Protein content per serving teaspoon red pepper flakes, or to taste
- Protein content per serving teaspoon celery seed
- 4 cups water (940 ml), divided
- 1 can (14.5 ounces, or 410 g) crushed tomatoes or tomato puree
- 1 head roasted garlic
- 2 tablespoons (30 g) prepared vegan pesto, plus more for garnish
- 2 cans (each 15 ounces, or 425 g) different kinds of white beans, drained and rinsed
- Protein content per serving cup (50 g)
- 1-inch (2.5 cm) pieces green beans
- Salt and pepper

Direction

- Heat the oil and salt in a large soup pot over medium heat. Add the onion, garlic, potatoes, carrots, and celery.
- Cook for 4 to 6 minutes, occasionally stirring, until the onions are translucent.
- Add the seasoning blend, red pepper flakes, and celery seed and stir for 2 minutes. Add 3 cups (705 ml) of the water and the crushed tomatoes.
- Combine the remaining 1 cup (235 ml) water and the roasted garlic in a blender.
- Process until smooth. Add to the soup mixture and bring to a boil. Reduce the heat to simmer and cook for 30 minutes.
- Stir in the pesto, beans, and green beans. Simmer for 15 minutes. Taste and adjust the seasonings. Serve each bowl with a dollop of pesto, if desired.

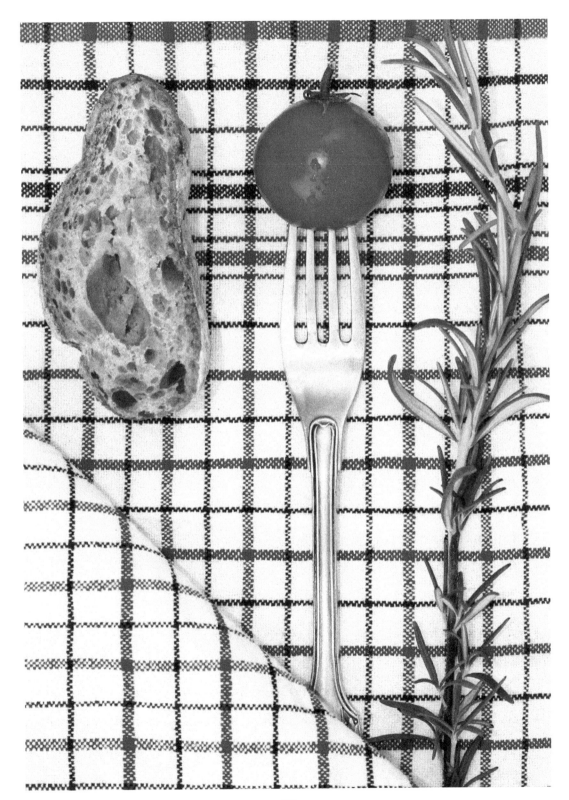

Plant Based Italian Style Special Recipes

- Easy Mushroom Pasta

Preparation Time: 5 Minutes

Cooking Time: 10 Minutes

Servings: 4

Ingredients:

- Chickpea Pasta (8 Oz.)
- Garlic Clove (2, Minced)
- Onion (1/4, Diced)
- Frozen Peas (1 C.)
- Vegan Butter (2 T.)
- Salt (to Taste)
- Bella Mushrooms (1 C., Sliced)
- Pepper (to taste)
- Italian Seasoning (1 t.)
- Optional: Fresh Parsley

Directions:

- The first step to making this quick and easy mushroom pasta will be cooking your pasta according to the directions in which are provided on the package.
- As the pasta cooks, you can also get out a skillet and set it above a moderate heat. Once it is warm, insert the butter and cook the peas, garlic, onion, and mushrooms for roughly five minutes.

- Once they are cooked through, you will want to plate your pasta and pour the mushroom mixture over the top.
- For a final touch, add some fresh parsley, and your meal will be ready.

Nutrition:

___

Calories: 260 | ***Carbs:*** 50g | ***Fats:*** 3g | ***Proteins:*** 10

- Creamed Avocado Pasta

Preparation Time: 5 Minutes

Cooking Time: 15 Minutes

Servings: 4

Ingredients:

- Whole-grain Pasta (3 C.)
- Olive Oil (1 T.)
- Spinach (1 C.)
- Garlic Cloves (2, Minced)
- Avocado (1)
- Pepper (1/4 t.)
- Lemon Juice (1 T.)
- Salt (to taste)
- Optional: Chili Flakes

Directions:

- First, cook your pasta according to the directions on the package.
- As the pasta cooks, it is time to make the avocado sauce! You can do this by taking out your blender and adding in the avocado, spinach, garlic, olive oil, lemon juice, and seasonings. Go ahead and blend this all together until it is smooth. If needed, you can add some water to make the sauce thinner.
- Next, you are going to want to plate your pasta and then serve the sauce over the top. For extra flavor, sprinkle some chili flakes before serving.

Calories: 300 |*Carbs:* 50g | *Fats:* 9g | *Proteins:* 10g

- Simple Hummus Pasta

Preparation Time: 5 Minutes

Cooking Time: 10 Minutes

Servings: 2

Ingredients:

- Whole Grain Pasta (2 C.)
- Salt (to taste)
- Cherry Tomatoes (1/2 C.)
- Hummus (1/2 C.)
- Pepper (to Taste)

Directions:

- As usual, begin this recipe by cooking the pasta to your liking.
- As the pasta cooks, prepare your tomatoes by chopping them in half.
- Once the pasta is cooked through, add it to a pan on top of low temperature and add in the tomatoes and the hummus. With everything in place, stir together for two or three minutes, and then your meal is set to be served!

Nutrition:

Calories: 300 |**Carbs:** 50g | **Fats:** 9g | **Proteins:** 10g

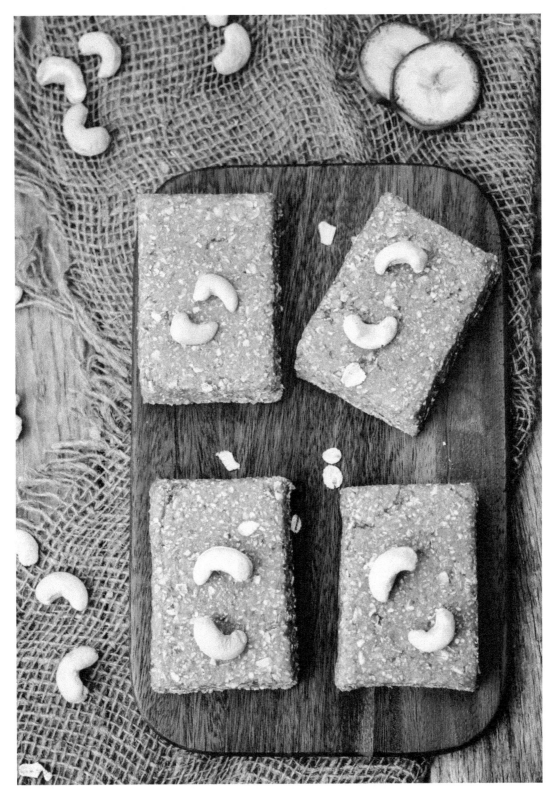

CHAPTER SIX

Dessert and Treats Recipes

- Simple Banana Cookies

Preparation Time: 5 Minutes

Cooking Time: 20 Minutes

Servings: 4

Ingredients:

- Peanut Butter (3 T.)
- Banana (2)
- Walnuts (1/4 C.)
- Rolled Oats (1 C.)

Directions:

- For a simple but delicious cookie, start by prepping the oven to 35As the oven warms up, take out your mixing bowl and first mash the bananas before adding in the oats.
- When you have folded the oats in, add in the walnuts and peanut butter before using your hands to layout small balls onto a baking sheet. Once this is set, pop the dish into the oven for fifteen minutes and bake your cookies.
- By the end of fifteen minutes, remove the dish from the oven and allow them to cool for five minutes before enjoying.

Nutrition:

Calories: 250 | ***Carbs:*** 30g | ***Fats:*** 10g | ***Proteins:*** 5g

- Basic Chocolate Cookies

Preparation Time: 5 Minutes

Cooking Time: 15 Minutes

Servings: 10

Ingredients:

- Cocoa Powder (1/2 C.)
- Almond Butter (1/2 C.)
- Bananas (2, Mashed)
- Salt (to Taste)

Directions:

- These chocolate cookies are a great way to get a touch of sweetness without overdoing the calories! To begin, prep the oven to 35
- As that heats, take out a mixing bowl so you can completely mash your bananas. When this is complete, carefully stir in the almond butter and the cocoa powder.
- Once your mixture is created, place tablespoons of the mix onto a lined cookie sheet and sprinkle a touch of salt over the top. When these are set, pop the dish into the oven for about fifteen minutes.
- Finally, remove the dish from the oven and cool before enjoying.

Nutrition:

Calories: 100 | *Carbs:* 10g | *Fats:* 5g | *Proteins:* 5g

- Quick Brownie Bites

Preparation Time: 10 Minutes

Cooking Time: 0 Minutes

Servings: 10

Ingredients:

- Cocoa Powder (1/4 C.)
- Medjool Dates (10)
- Vanilla Extract (1 t.)
- Walnut Halves (1 ½ C.)
- Water (1 T.)

Directions:

- to be honest, who isn't guilty of eating cookie dough raw? Now, you can do it on purpose! To begin this recipe, you will first need to get out a food processor so you can break down the Medjool dates. Once these are broken down, add in the rest of the ingredients and blend until combined.
- Now that you have your batter, roll it into small balls, and your dessert is ready in an instant!

Nutrition:

Calories: 150 | **Carbs:** 15g | **Fats:** 10g | **Proteins:** 5g

- Peach Crisp

Preparation Time: 5 Minutes

Cooking Time: 15 Minutes

Servings: 2

Ingredients:

- Rolled Oats (2 T.)
- Flour (1 t.)
- Brown Sugar (2 T.)
- Peaches (2, Diced)
- Sugar (1 t.)
- Coconut Oil (3 t.)
- Flour (3 t.)

Directions:

- This recipe is built for two! You can begin by prepping the oven to 375 and getting out two small baking dishes.
- As the oven begins to warm, take one of the mixing bowls and toss the peach pieces with the sugar, cinnamon, and a teaspoon of flour. When this is set, pour the peaches into a baking dish.
- In the other bowl, mix together the three teaspoons of flour with the oats and the sugar. Once these are blended, pour in coconut oil and continue mixing. Now that you have your crumble, place it over the peaches in the baking dish.

- Finally, you are going to pop the dish into the oven for fifteen minutes or until the top is a nice golden color. If it looks finished, remove and cool before slicing your dessert up.

Calories: 110 | *Carbs:* 20g | *Fats:* 5g | *Proteins:* 2g

- Chocolate Dessert Dip

Preparation Time: 10 Minutes

Cooking Time: 0 Minutes

Servings: 6

Ingredients:

- Date Paste (1/2 C.)
- Cocoa (1/4 C.)
- Cashew Butter (1/2 C.)

Directions:

- Do you need to whip up dessert quickly? This is an excellent recipe to have on hand, especially if you want to impress your guests! All you have to do is place the three ingredients into a food processor and mix until blended.
- Simply place the dip into a serving dish, and you are ready to go.

Nutrition:

Calories: 150 | ***Carbs:*** 15g | ***Fats:*** 10g | ***Proteins:*** 5g

- Lemon Coconut Cookies

Preparation Time: 15 Minutes

Cooking Time: 0 Minutes

Servings: 4

Ingredients:

- Coconut Flour (1/3 C.)
- Shredded Coconut (1 ½ C.)
- Agave (6 T.)
- Almond Flour (1 ½ C.)
- Lemon Zest (1 T.)
- Lemon Juice (4 T.)
- Coconut Oil (1 T.)
- Vanilla Extract (2 t.)
- Salt (to Taste)

Directions:

- If you enjoy dessert but are looking for something that isn't chocolate, this recipe will be perfect for you! To make these incredible cookies, you will want to place all of the ingredients from the list, minus the shredded coconut, into the food processor, and blend until you have created a dough.
- Once your dough is set, take your hands and roll the dough into small, bite-sized balls.
- As a final touch, roll the balls in your shredded coconut and then place into

the fridge for twenty minutes. After this time has passed, go ahead and enjoy your dessert!

Nutrition:

Calories: 450 | *Carbs:* 30g | *Fats:* 20g | *Proteins:* 10g

- Watermelon Pizza

Preparation Time: 15 Minutes

Cooking Time: 0 Minutes

Servings: 4

Ingredients:

- Watermelon (1, Sliced)
- Banana (1, Sliced)
- Blueberries (1 C.)
- Coconut Flakes (1/2 C.)
- Chopped Walnuts (1/4 C.)

Directions:

- This dessert is pretty simple, but it can be a lot of fun to make and eat if you have kids in the house! You will begin this recipe by taking the watermelon and chopping it up to look like pizza slices.
- When the watermelon slices are set, you can then add the chopped fruit on top of the watermelon, followed by any chopped nuts and coconut flakes. For this recipe, we chose to use bananas and blueberries, but you can use any fruit that you like!
- Just like that, you have watermelon pizza for dessert!

Nutrition:

Calories: 50 | *Carbs:* 10g | *Fats:* 3g | *Proteins:* 1g

- Sweet & spicy snack mix

Preparation time: 5 minutes

Cooking time: 18 minutes

Servings: 20

Ingredients:

- 4 cups mixed vegetable sticks
- ½ cup whole almonds
- 2 cups corn square cereal
- 2 cups oat cereal, toasted
- 1 ¾ cups pretzel sticks
- 1 teaspoon packed brow n sugar
- 1 teaspoon paprika
- ½ teaspoon chili powder
- ½ teaspoon ground cumin
- ¼ teaspoon cayenne pepper
- Salt to taste
- Cooking spray

Directions:

- Preheat your oven to 300 degrees f.
- In a roasting pan, add the vegetable sticks, almonds, corn and oat cereals and pretzel sticks.

- In a bowl, mix the rest of the ingredients.
- Coat the cereal mixture with cooking spray.
- Sprinkle spice mixture on top of the cereals.
- Bake in the oven for 18 minutes.
- Store in an airtight container for up to 7 days.

- Carrot & peppers with hummus

Preparation time: 5 minutes

Cooking time: 0 minute

Serving: 1

Ingredients:

- ½ green bell pepper, sliced
- 2 carrots, sliced into sticks
- 3 tablespoons hummus

Directions:

- Arrange carrot and pepper slices in a food container.
- Place hummus in a smaller food container and add to the big food container beside the carrot and peppers.

- Snickerdoodle Energy Balls

Preparation Time: 10 Minutes

Cooking Time: 0 Minutes

Servings: 20

Ingredients:

- Medjool Dates (1 C.)
- Ground Cinnamon (2 t.)
- Cashews (1 C.)
- Vanilla Extract (1/4 t.)
- Almonds (1/2 C.)
- Salt (to Taste)

Directions:

- These little snacks are great op hand because they offer a boost of protein and are easy to grab on the go! To start out, you will want to place your Medjool dates into a food processor and blend until the Medjool dates become soft and sticky.
- Next, you can add the nuts and seasoning along with the vanilla extract and blend until completely combined.
- Now that you have your dough use your hand to create bite-sized balls and place onto a plate. You can enjoy them instantly or place them in the fridge for thirty minutes and wait for them to harden up a bit.

- Baked Carrot Chips

Preparation Time: 10 Minutes

Cooking Time: 30 Minutes

Servings: 8

Ingredients:

- Olive Oil (1/4 C.)
- Ground Cinnamon (1 t.)
- Ground Cumin (1 t.)
- Salt (to Taste)
- Carrots (3 Pounds)

Directions:

- As you begin a plant-based diet, you may find yourself craving something crunchy. This recipe offers the best of both worlds by giving you a crunch and something nutritious to snack on. You can begin this recipe by heating your oven to 425 and setting up a baking sheet with some parchment paper.
- Next, you will want to chop the top off each carrot and slice the carrot up paper-thin. You can complete this task by using a knife, but it typically is easier if you have a mandolin slicer.
- With your carrot slices all prepared, next, you will want to toss them in a small bowl with the cinnamon, cumin, olive oil, and a touch of salt. When the carrot slices are well coated, go ahead and lay them across your baking sheet.
- Finally, you are going to pop the carrots into the oven for fifteen minutes.

After this time, you may notice that the edges are going to start to curl and get crispy. At this point, remove the dish from the oven and flip all of the chips over. Place the dish back into the oven for six or seven minutes, and then your chips will be set!

- Sweet Cinnamon Chips

Preparation Time: 5 Minutes

Cooking Time: 15 Minutes

Servings: 5

Ingredients:

- Whole Wheat Tortillas (10)
- Ground Cinnamon (1 t.)
- Sugar (3 T.)
- Olive Oil (2 C.)

Directions:

- If you are looking for a snack that is sweet and simple, these chips should do the trick! You are going to want to start out by getting out a small bowl so you can mix the cinnamon and sugar together. When this is complete, set it to the side.
- Next, you will want to get out your frying pan and bring the olive oil to a soft simmer. While the oil gets to a simmer, take some time to slice your tortillas up into wedges. When these are set, carefully place them into your simmering olive oil and cook for about two minutes on each side, or until golden.
- Once the chips are all set, pat them down with a paper towel and then generously coat each chip with the cinnamon mixture you made earlier. After that, your chips will be set for your enjoyment.

- Creamy Avocado Hummus

Preparation Time: 5 Minutes

Cooking Time: 0 Minutes

Servings: 4

Ingredients:

- Olive Oil (1 T.)
- Avocado (1)
- White Beans (1 Can)
- Cayenne Pepper (1/4 t.)
- Lime Juice (2 t.)

Directions:

1. When you are looking for something smooth and creamy to dip your vegetables or chips in, this is the perfect recipe to give a try!
2. All you will have to do is place the ingredients from the list above into the food processor and process until smooth.
3. Place the avocado hummus into a serving bowl, and you are ready to dip.

- Cauliflower Popcorn

Preparation Time: 10 Minutes

Cooking Time: 0 Minutes

Servings: 4

Ingredients:

- Olive Oil (2 T.)
- Chili Powder (2 t.)
- Cumin (2 t.)
- Nutritional Yeast (1 T.)
- Cauliflower (1 Head)
- Salt (to Taste)

Directions:

- Before you begin making this recipe, you will want to take a few moments to cut your cauliflower into bite-sized pieces, like popcorn!
- Once your cauliflower is set, place it into a mixing bowl and coat with the olive oil. Once coated properly, add in the nutritional yeast, salt, and the rest of the spices.
- You can enjoy your snack immediately or place into a dehydrator at 115 for 8 hours. By doing this, it will make the cauliflower crispy! You can really enjoy it either way.

- Banana and Strawberry Oat Bars

Preparation Time: 10 Minutes

Cooking Time: 1 Hour

Servings: 5

Ingredients:

- Rolled Oats (2 C.)
- Chia Seeds (2 T.)
- Maple Syrup (1/4 C.)
- Strawberries (2 C.)
- Vanilla Extract (2 t.)
- Bananas (2, Mashed)
- Maple Syrup (2 T.)
- Baking Powder (1 t.)

Directions:

- These oat bars take a few different steps, but they are a great snack to have when you are short on time! You are going to start off by making the strawberry jam for the bars. You can do this by placing the strawberries and two tablespoons of maple syrup into a pan and place it over medium heat.
- After about fifteen minutes, the strawberries should be releasing their liquid and will come to a boil. You will want to boil for an additional ten minutes.
- As a final touch for the jam, gently stir in the one teaspoon of the vanilla extract and the chia seeds. Be sure that you continue stirring for an

additional five minutes before removing from the heat and setting to the side.

- Now, it is time to make the bars! You can start this part out by prepping the oven to 375 and getting together a baking dish and lining it with parchment paper.

- Next, you are going to want to add one cup of your oats into a food processor and blend until they look like flour. At this point, you can pour the oats into a mixing bowl and place in the rest of the oats along with the baking powder.

- Once these ingredients are blended well, throw in the other teaspoon of vanilla, maple syrup, and your mashed bananas. As you mix everything together, you will notice that you are now forming a dough.

- When you are ready to assemble the bars, you will want to take half of the mixture and press it into the bottom of your baking dish and carefully spoon the jam over the surface. Once these are set, add the rest of the dough over the top and press down ever so slightly.

- Finally, you are going to want to place the dish into the oven and cook for about thirty minutes. By the end of this time, the top of your bars should be golden, and you can remove the dish from the oven. Allow the bars to cool slightly before slicing and enjoying.

- PB Cookie Dough Balls

Preparation Time: 10 Minutes

Cooking Time: 0 Minutes

Servings: 8

Ingredients:

- Whole Wheat Flour (2 C.)
- Maple Syrup (1 C.)
- Peanuts (1/2 C.)
- Peanut Butter (1 C.)
- Rolled Oats (1/2 C.)

Directions:

- Is this recipe a snack or dessert? That is completely up to you! To start this recipe, you will want to get out a large mixing bowl and combine all of the ingredients from the list above.
- Once they are well blended, take your hands and carefully roll the dough into bite-sized balls before you enjoy! For easier handling, you will want to place the balls into the fridge for about twenty minutes before enjoying.

- Almond Millet Chews

Preparation Time: 15 Minutes

Cooking Time: 0 Minutes

Servings: 10

Ingredients:

- Millet (1 C.)
- Almond Butter (1/2 C.)
- Raisins (1/4 C.)
- Brown Rice Syrup (1/4 C.)

Directions:

- This dessert is perfect for when you want something small after dinner. You will want to begin by melting the almond butter in the microwave for about twenty seconds.
- When this step is complete, place it into a mixing bowl with the brown rice syrup, raisins, and millets.
- Once everything is blended well, use your hands to roll balls and place onto a plate.
- If needed, you can add a touch more syrup to keep everything together. Place into the fridge for twenty minutes and then enjoy your dessert.

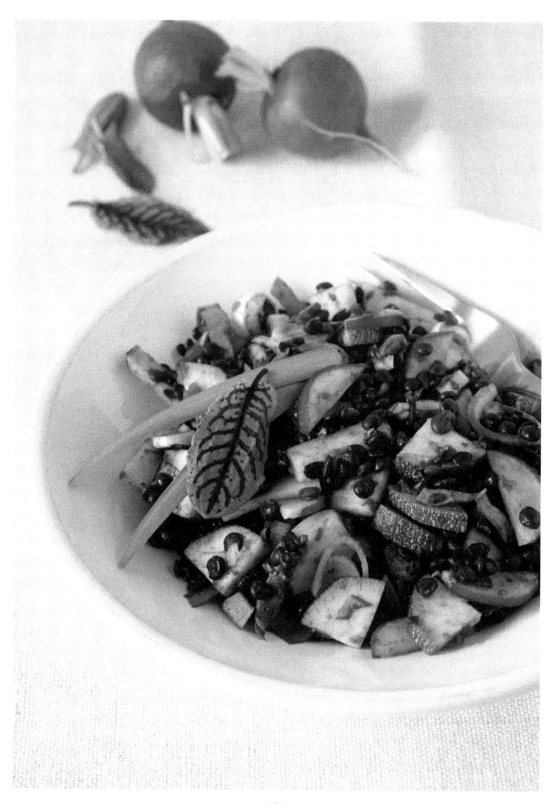

Snacks and Salads Recipes

- Lentil Radish Salad

Preparation time: 15 minutes

Cooking Time: 0 minutes

Servings: 3

Ingredients:

Dressing:

- 1 tbsp. extra virgin olive oil
- 1 tbsp. lemon juice
- 1 tbsp. maple syrup
- 1 tbsp. water
- ½ tbsp. sesame oil
- 1 tbsp. miso paste, yellow or white
- ¼ tsp. salt
- ¼ tsp Pepper

Salad:

- ½ cup dry chickpeas
- ¼ cup dry green or brown lentils
- 1 14-oz. pack of silken tofu
- 5 cups mixed greens, fresh or frozen
- 2 radishes, thinly sliced

- ½ cup cherry tomatoes, halved
- ¼ cup roasted sesame seeds

Directions:

- Prepare the chickpeas according to the method.
- Prepare the lentils according to the method.
- Put all the ingredients for the dressing in a blender or food processor. Mix on low until smooth, while adding water until it reaches the desired consistency.
- Add salt, pepper (to taste), and optionally more water to the dressing; set aside.
- Cut the tofu into bite-sized cubes.
- Combine the mixed greens, tofu, lentils, chickpeas, radishes, and tomatoes in a large bowl.
- Add the dressing and mix everything until it is coated evenly.
- Top with the optional roasted sesame seeds, if desired.
- Refrigerate before serving and enjoy, or, store for later!

Nutrition:

Calories 621, Total Fat 19.6g, Saturated Fat 2.8g, Cholesterol 0mg, Sodium 996mg, Total Carbohydrate 82.7g, Dietary Fiber 26.1g, Total Sugars 20.7g, Protein 31.3g, Vitamin D 0mcg, Calcium 289mg, Iron 9mg, Potassium 1370mg

- Shaved Brussel Sprout Salad

Preparation time: 25 minutes

Cooking time: 0 minutes

Servings: 4

Ingredients:

Dressing:

- 1 tbsp. brown mustard
- 1 tbsp. maple syrup
- 2 tbsp. apple cider vinegar
- 2 tbsp. extra virgin olive oil
- ½ tbsp. garlic minced

Salad:

- ½ cup dry red kidney beans
- ¼ cup dry chickpeas
- 2 cups Brussel sprouts
- 1 cup purple onion
- 1 small sour apple
- ½ cup slivered almonds, crushed
- ½ cup walnuts, crushed
- ½ cup cranberries, dried
- ¼ tsp Salt
- ¼ tsp pepper

Directions:

- Prepare the beans according to the method.
- Combine all dressing ingredients in a bowl and stir well until combined.
- Refrigerate the dressing for up to one hour before serving.
- Using a grater, mandolin, or knife to thinly slice each Brussel sprout. Repeat this with the apple and onion.
- Take a large bowl to mix the chickpeas, beans, sprouts, apples, onions, cranberries, and nuts.
- Drizzle the cold dressing over the salad to coat.
- Serve with salt and pepper to taste, or, store for later!

Nutrition:

Calories 432, Total Fat 23.5g, Saturated Fat 2.2g, Cholesterol 0mg, Sodium 197mg, Total Carbohydrate 45.3g, Dietary Fiber 12.4g, Total Sugars 14g, Protein 15.9g, Vitamin D 0mcg, Calcium 104mg, Iron 4mg, Potassium 908mg

- Colorful Protein Power Salad

Preparation time: 20 minutes

Cooking Time: 0 minutes

Servings: 2

Ingredients:

- ½ cup dry quinoa
- 2 cups dry navy beans
- 1 green onion, chopped
- 2 tsp. garlic, minced
- 3 cups green or purple cabbage, chopped
- 4 cups kale, fresh or frozen, chopped
- 1 cup shredded carrot, chopped
- 2 tbsp. extra virgin olive oil
- 1 tsp. lemon juice
- ¼ tsp Salt
- ¼ tsp pepper

Directions:

- Prepare the quinoa according to the recipe.
- Prepare the beans according to the method.
- Heat up 1 tablespoon of the olive oil in a frying pan over medium heat.
- Add the chopped green onion, garlic, and cabbage, and sauté for 2-3 minutes.

- Add the kale, the remaining 1 tablespoon of olive oil, and salt. Lower the heat and cover until the greens have wilted, around 5 minutes. Remove the pan from the stove and set aside.
- Take a large bowl and mix the remaining ingredients with the kale and cabbage mixture once it has cooled down. Add more salt and pepper to taste.
- Mix until everything is distributed evenly.
- Serve topped with a dressing, or, store for later!

Nutrition:

Calories 1100, Total Fat 19.9g, Saturated Fat 2.7g, Cholesterol 0mg, Sodium 420mg, Total Carbohydrate 180.8g, Dietary Fiber 60.1g, Total Sugars 14.4g, Protein 58.6g, Vitamin D 0mcg, Calcium 578mg, Iron 16mg, Potassium 3755mg

- Edamame & Ginger Citrus Salad

Preparation time: 15 minutes

Cooking Time: 0 minutes

Servings: 3

Ingredients:

Dressing:

- ¼ cup orange juice
- 1 tsp. lime juice
- ½ tbsp. maple syrup
- ½ tsp. ginger, finely minced
- ½ tbsp. sesame oil
- Salad:
- ½ cup dry green lentils
- 2 cups carrots, shredded
- 4 cups kale, fresh or frozen, chopped
- 1 cup edamame, shelled
- 1 tablespoon roasted sesame seeds
- 2 tsp. mint, chopped
- Salt and pepper to taste
- 1 small avocado, peeled, pitted, diced

Directions:

- Prepare the lentils according to the method.

- Combine the orange and lime juices, maple syrup, and ginger in a small bowl. Mix with a whisk while slowly adding the sesame oil.
- Add the cooked lentils, carrots, kale, edamame, sesame seeds, and mint to a large bowl.
- Add the dressing and stir well until all the ingredients are coated evenly.
- Store or serve topped with avocado and an additional sprinkle of mint.

Nutrition:

Calories 507, Total Fat 23.1g, Saturated Fat 4g, Cholesterol 0mg, Sodium 303mg, Total Carbohydrate 56.8g, Dietary Fiber 21.6g, Total Sugars 8.4g, Protein 24.6g, Vitamin D 0mcg, Calcium 374mg, Iron 8mg, Potassium 1911mg

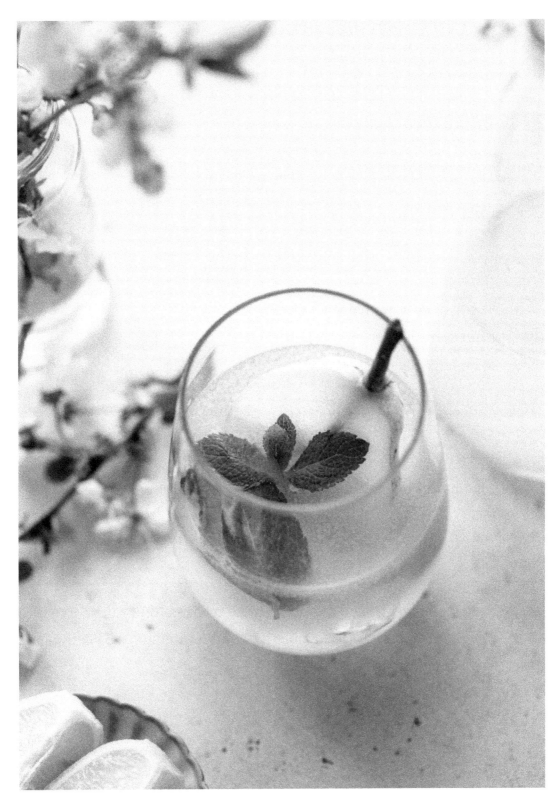

DRINKS AND SMOOTHIES RECIPEE

- Pear Lemonade

Preparation time: 5 minutes

Cooking time: 30 minutes

Serving: 2

Ingredients:

- ½ cup of pear, peeled and diced
- 1 cup of freshly squeezed lemon juice
- ½ cup of chilled water

Directions:

- Add all the ingredients into a blender and pulse until it has all been combined. The pear does make the lemonade frothy, but this will settle.
- Place in the refrigerator to cool and then serve.

Tips:

1. Keep stored in a sealed container in the refrigerator for up to four days.
2. Pop the fresh lemon in the microwave for ten minutes before juicing, you can extract more juice if you do this.

- Colorful Infused Water

Preparation time: 5 minutes

Cooking time: 1 hour

Serving: 8

Ingredients:

- 1 cup of strawberries, fresh or frozen
- 1 cup of blueberries, fresh or frozen
- 1 tablespoon of baobab powder
- 1 cup of ice cubes
- 4 cups of sparkling water

Directions:

1. In a large water jug, add in the sparkling water, ice cubes, and baobab powder. Give it a good stir.
2. Add in the strawberries and blueberries and cover the infused water, store in the refrigerator for one hour before serving.

Tips:

1. Store for 12 hours for optimum taste and nutritional benefits.
2. Instead of using strawberries and blueberries, add slices of lemon and six mint leaves, one cup of mangoes or cherries, or half a cup of leafy greens such as kale and/or spinach.

- Hibiscus Tea

Preparation time: 1 Minute

Cooking time: 5 minutes

Serving: 2

Ingredients:

- 1 tablespoon of raisins, diced
- 6 Almonds, raw and unsalted
- ½ teaspoon of hibiscus powder
- 2 cups of water

Directions:

- Bring the water to a boil in a small saucepan, add in the hibiscus powder and raisins. Give it a good stir, cover and let simmer for a further two minutes.
- Strain into a teapot and serve with a side helping of almonds.

Tips:

1. As an alternative to this tea, do not strain it and serve with the raisin pieces still swirling around in the teacup.
2. You could also serve this tea chilled for those hotter days.
3. Double or triple the recipe to provide you with iced-tea to enjoy during the week without having to make a fresh pot each time.

- Lemon and Rosemary Iced Tea

Preparation time: 5 minutes

Cooking time: 10 minutes

Serving: 4

Ingredients:

- 4 cups of water
- 4 earl grey tea bags
- ¼ cup of sugar
- 2 lemons
- 1 sprig of rosemary

Directions:

- Peel the two lemons and set the fruit aside.
- In a medium saucepan, over medium heat combines the water, sugar, and lemon peels. Bring this to a boil.
- Remove from the heat and place the rosemary and tea into the mixture. Cover the saucepan and steep for five minutes.
- Add the juice of the two peeled lemons to the mixture, strain, chill, and serve.

Tips:

1. Skip the sugar and use honey to taste.
2. Do not squeeze the tea bags as they can cause the tea to become bitter.

- Peanut Butter Smoothie

Preparation time: 5 minutes

Cooking time: 5 minutes

Serving: 2

Ingredients:

- 1 and ½ cups of almond, soy or coconut milk, unsweetened
- 2 bananas, peeled and frozen 12 hours before use
- ½ teaspoon of vanilla essence
- 1 tablespoon of cocoa powder
- 2 tablespoons of peanut butter

Directions:

- Add all the ingredients into a blender, pulse until smooth and serve.

Tips:

- You may substitute the peanut butter for any other nut butter.

- Cinnamon Smoothie

Preparation time: 5 minutes

Cooking time: 5 minutes

Serving: 2

Ingredients:

- 1 and ½ cups of almond, soy or coconut milk, unsweetened
- 2 bananas, peeled and frozen 12 hours before use
- ½ teaspoon of vanilla essence
- ½ teaspoon of cinnamon
- ½ cup of oats, rolled
- 3 dated, pitted and halved
- Directions:
- Add all the ingredients into a blender, pulse until smooth and serve.

Tips:

- Feel free to add more cinnamon or oats for a more filling smoothie.

- Green Smoothie

Preparation time: 5 minutes

Cooking time: 5 minutes

Serving: 2

Ingredients:

- 2 cups of almond milk
- 1 banana, peeled and frozen 12 hours before use
- 1 cup of spinach
- ½ an avocado
- 2 tablespoons hemp hearts
- 2 tablespoons of chia seeds

Directions:

- Add all the ingredients into a blender, pulse until smooth and serve.
- Tips:
- You may substitute the almond milk for another milk of your choice.

- Green Piña Colada Smoothie

Preparation time: 5 minutes

Cooking time: 5 minutes

Serving: 2

Ingredients:

- 2 cups of light coconut milk
- 1 banana, peeled and frozen 12 hours before use
- 1 cup of pineapple, frozen
- 1 teaspoon of vanilla extract

Directions:

- Add all the ingredients into a blender, pulse until smooth and serve.

Tips:

- For a creamier option, opt to use 1 cup of light coconut milk with 1 cup of full-fat coconut milk.

- Ginger and Berry Smoothie

Preparation time: 5 minutes

Cooking time: 5 minutes

Serving: 2

Ingredients:

- 2 cups of almond milk
- 1 knob of ginger
- 1 cup of strawberries, frozen
- 1 cup of raspberries, frozen
- 1 cup of cauliflower, steam before use in recipe

Directions:

- Add all the ingredients into a blender, pulse until smooth and serve.

Tips:

- The reason the cauliflower is steamed before use is because it is easier on digestion.
- Frozen fruits thicken a smoothie more than fresh fruits.

- Lime and Raspberry Smoothie

Preparation time: 5 minutes

Cooking time: 5 minutes

Serving: 2

Ingredients:

- 1 cup of water
- 1 banana, peeled and frozen 12 hours before use
- 1 cup of raspberries, frozen
- 1 teaspoon of coconut oil
- 2 teaspoons of lime juice
- 1 teaspoon of sweetener of your choice

Directions:

- Add all the ingredients into a blender, pulse until smooth and serve.

Tips:

- Add blocks of ice to the blender for added texture.

- Avocado, Blueberry, and Chia Smoothie

Preparation time: 5 minutes

Cooking time: 5 minutes

Serving: 2

Ingredients:

- 2 cups of almond milk
- 2 cups of blueberries, frozen
- 1 avocado, peeled and pitted
- 2 dates, pitted
- 2 tablespoons of flax or chia
- ½ teaspoon of vanilla extract

Directions:

- Add the blueberries, avocado, dates, chia or flax, and vanilla extract to a blender. Pulse until smooth.
- Add in the almond milk and pulse until combined with the rest of the mixture, serve.

Tips:

- Substitute the almond milk for coconut milk if you'd prefer.

- Coconut, Raspberry, and Quinoa Smoothie

Preparation time: 5 minutes

Cooking time: 5 minutes

Serving: 2

Ingredients:

- 2 cups of coconut milk
- 2 cups of raspberries, frozen
- 4 tablespoons of goji berries
- 2 dates, pitted
- 1 cup of quinoa, cooked
- 4 tablespoons of coconut, shredded

Directions:

- Add all the ingredients into a blender, pulse until smooth and serve.

Tips:

- Substitute the coconut milk for almond milk for a different taste.

CONCLUSION

It was an awesome journey taking you through the varieties of plant-based recipe which you might not have known before, so as to spice up your vegan lifestyle.

If you try all these recipes listed in here, you are going to have an amazing lifestyle as a plant-based diet personnel and apart from that you will live a healthier life than before when you've not chosen plant-based diet. Also, one more secret, you can try this diet with family and friends, by inviting them over for dinner and show them what they've been missing in terms of mouthwatering recipe and the benefits they are missing by not opting for plant-based diet. Keep enjoying and exploring the more about this diet.

Lightning Source UK Ltd.
Milton Keynes UK
UKHW051028250621
386136UK00002B/4